How to Date Older Men

Unveiling the Beauty of Age Gap Romance

Michelle Mann

Copyright © 2023 by Michelle Mann

All rights reserved.

No portion of this book may be reproduced in any form without written permission from the publisher or author, except as permitted by U.S. copyright law.

Contents

1. Introduction   1
2. Understanding the Allure   4
3. Communication is Key   21
4. Navigating the Financial Landscape   37
5. Bridging Cultural and Social Gaps   54
6. Planning for the Future   70
7. Intimacy and Physical Connection   85
8. Building Strong Foundations   100
9. Celebrating Age-Gap Love Stories   128
10. Conclusion   144

Chapter One

Introdution

Ah, the captivating dance of two souls, unfettered by the conventions of time. There's something both timeless and profoundly beautiful about age-gap romances. It's like a melody where two different instruments, each from a distinct epoch, come together to create a symphony that resonates through the ages. This dance, as with any, has its steps, its rhythms, and its nuances—each just waiting to be explored.

Setting the Stage: The Allure of Age-Gap Romances

When we speak of romance and love, what often comes to mind? A shared glance, a gentle touch, an intimate conversation under a canopy of stars. Love, in its purest form, transcends age. It's the shared laughter, the mutual respect, the joy of finding someone who understands your very essence. With older men, there often comes a certain level of maturity, wisdom, and understanding—a gravitas molded by experiences, triumphs, and tribulations. This depth can offer a sense of security, a grounding, that's incredibly alluring. It's not just about the years but the stories, lessons, and dreams that come with them.

And for the young at heart, there's a refreshing zeal, a vibrant pulse of life that offers a rejuvenation, a chance to relive and rethink. When these two worlds collide, the potential for a rich, fulfilling relationship is boundless.

Demystifying Misconceptions: Common Myths About Dating Older Men

But, like a rose with its thorns, this unique love comes intertwined with societal misconceptions. Whispered conversations, raised eyebrows, the unasked questions hanging in the air—dating older men often brings baggage of myths. Some believe it's all about financial security, while others might cheekily suggest it's a fleeting phase or a rebellion. The truth? As diverse as the stories of the stars in the night sky. Every age-gap relationship has its narrative, its heartbeat. It's crucial to recognize these myths for what they are—simply stereotypes, not the rule. Throughout this journey, we'll delve deeper into dispelling these myths, paving the way for understanding and acceptance.

What to Expect in the Guide: An Overview of the Journey Ahead

Embarking on this exploration, you'll be gently guided through the verdant valleys and towering peaks of age-gap relationships. From understanding the very allure of dating older men, and navigating the intricacies of communication, to planning a shared future, this guide seeks to be your compass. Think of it as a heart-to-heart chat with a dear friend, over a warm cup of tea, sharing tales, advice, and little nuggets of wisdom. Together, we'll unravel the fabric of age-gap love, stitch by stitch, weaving a tapestry that's as vibrant as it is insightful.

So, settle in, dear reader, and let's embark on this heartwarming journey together. Embrace the dance, celebrate the romance, and unveil the beauty of love that knows no age.

Chapter Two

Understanding the Allure

"Age does not protect you from love, but love, to some extent, protects you from age." – Jeanne Moreau

Love is a mystifying, beautiful enigma. Its patterns are as varied as the stars that grace our night sky. Each romance is unique; each connection is profound. Among the myriad forms love takes, age-gap romances have their distinct charm—a mesmerizing waltz of youthful vigor and timeless wisdom. But what truly lies behind this allure? Let's delve deeper and unravel the magic.

1. The Timeless Charm of Maturity:

- **Wisdom's allure**: Older men often bring a wealth of experiences to the table. Their stories, filled with life's trials and tribulations, paint a vivid tapestry that can captivate a younger heart. Their perspectives, molded by time, offer a depth that's both comforting and enlightening.

- **Stability's embrace**: With age often comes a sense of stability, both emotional and financial. This grounded presence can be a haven in the unpredictable whirlwind of life.

- **Gentle guidance**: An older partner's seasoned insights can offer guidance in life's labyrinth, nurturing growth and fostering understanding.

2. The Vibrancy of Youth:

- **Renewed vigor**: Younger individuals breathe fresh life into a relationship. Their zest for life, their curiosity, and their ever-evolving dreams can rekindle a fire in older souls, inspiring them to see the world through newer, more vibrant lenses.

- **A fresh perspective**: The world changes with each passing day, and so does our understanding of it. Younger partners introduce new thoughts, cultures, and trends, leading to stimulating conversations and shared discoveries.

- **Playful adventures**: Youth is synonymous with adventure. The eagerness to explore, to challenge norms, and to embrace spontaneity can add an exciting dynamic to the relationship.

3. A Symphony of Differences:

- **Complementary strengths**: Age-gap relationships often thrive on the yin-yang principle. Where one might have patience, the other brings passion; where one offers security, the other introduces adventure.

- **Shared growth**: Differences pave the way for learning. By embracing each other's unique viewpoints, couples can evolve together, enriching their shared journey.

- **Cherished moments**: The fusion of two worlds creates memories that are uniquely theirs—like watching an old classic film for the first time or introducing a partner to the wonders of modern tech.

4. Deep Emotional Connections:

- **Beyond the superficial**: Age-gap romances often delve deeper than mere physical attraction. They are rooted in mutual respect, shared values, and emotional depth.

- **Embracing vulnerabilities**: With the blend of youth and age, partners can create a safe space where vulnerabilities are not just shared but cherished, leading to profound emotional bonds.

- **Unwavering support**: Whether it's the support of a mature partner during life's challenges or the younger one's unwavering faith in dreams, such relationships are pillars of strength for each other.

5. Defying Societal Norms:

- **A testament to courage**: Choosing an age-gap relationship often requires defying societal expectations, and showcasing the couple's courage and commitment to their love.

- **Fostering acceptance**: By living their truth, age-gap couples pave the way for broader acceptance of diverse relationships, inspiring others.

- **Building resilience**: Navigating societal perceptions can fortify the relationship, making it resilient to external pressures.

In the realm of love, age is but a number. The allure of age-gap romances lies not in the years between partners but in the shared moments, the mingling dreams, and the harmonious dance of two souls. It's a world where hearts find their rhythm, not in the tick of a clock, but in the beats of shared experiences. As we journey further, let's celebrate this enchanting allure, cherishing its nuances and understanding its depths.

***

The Timeless Appeal – A Journey Through Ages and Emotions

Ever paused to think about how tales of age-gap romances have always been intertwined with the fabric of history? From fables to real-life stories, age-mixed relationships have captivated hearts and minds alike. They are a testament to love's ability to transcend the linear confines of time. Let's embark on a journey to understand the allure that has persisted through the ages.

The Historical Context of Age-Gap Relationships:

- **Ancient allure**: Historical texts, artifacts, and literature from ancient civilizations, like Egypt and Greece, carry tales of age-gap relationships, both in the royal circles and among common folks. These stories often depicted relationships with older men as symbols of power, wisdom, and protection. Think of Cleopatra and Julius Caesar or Antony – these relationships were as much about political alliance as they were about genuine affection and respect.

- **Medieval sentiments**: In medieval times, age-gap marriages often had socio-economic implications. Families sought older, established men for their young daughters, hoping for stability and protection. But amidst these strategic alliances, there were genuine tales of love, passion, and deep connections.

- **Modern manifestations**: With changing societal norms and the pursuit of personal happiness over convention, age-gap relationships in modern times are seen more as personal choices. They are celebrated in literature, films, and pop culture, highlighting the genuine emotional bonds over societal constructs.

Mature Men's Appeal to Younger Women:

- **A rock in the storm**: Older men often provide a sense of stability and security that's deeply appealing. Their life experiences have given them a perspective and maturity that can act as an anchor in the turbulent seas of life.

- **The allure of wisdom**: With years comes wisdom, and with wisdom comes a depth of understanding. This can lead to meaningful conversations, shared learnings, and a bond that goes beyond mere physical attraction.

- **Gentle mentorship**: An older partner often becomes a guide, a mentor in the journey of life. They offer insights from their experiences, helping navigate challenges with a balanced viewpoint.

The Emotional Depth of Age-Mixed Relationships:

- **Beyond the superficial**: Age-gap relationships, owing to the differences in life stages, often prioritize emotional connection over fleeting physical attractions. This foundation leads to a richer, deeper bond that stands the test of time.

- **Shared growth**: Such relationships provide a unique opportunity for both partners to grow. The younger partner benefits from the older one's experiences, while the older partner gets a fresh, youthful perspective on life.

- **A safe haven**: The blend of youth's passion with age's wisdom creates a safe space. Vulnerabilities are cherished, emotions are deeply understood, and what results is a relationship where both partners feel valued, respected, and deeply loved.

The timeless appeal of age-gap romances is not just a product of societal constructs but a genuine testament to love's ability to find its match beyond the boundaries of age. It's a dance of youthful energy and mature understanding, creating a symphony that's been celebrated through the annals of history and continues to captivate hearts today.

***

Beyond Physical Attraction

Physical attraction might be the spark that ignites many romances, but for a relationship to thrive, especially one with an age difference, there needs to be a deeper, more robust foundation. Age-gap relationships offer a plethora of intangible benefits that go beyond the superficial. It's not just about the fleeting rush of hormones but the intertwining of souls, dreams, and shared journeys. Let's explore the facets that form this deep-rooted foundation.

Emotional Stability and Experience:

- **A seasoned perspective**: Older partners have journeyed through life's ups and downs, faced challenges, and celebrated its triumphs. This seasoned perspective allows them to approach relationship hurdles with calmness, understanding, and maturity.

- **Navigating emotional landscapes**: With years come the wisdom to recognize and understand emotions better. This ability to navigate emotional landscapes can lead to a harmonious relationship where both partners feel heard and valued.

- **Building trust**: Experience in past relationships or life challenges often instills the value of trust. An older partner's understanding of trust's importance can create a solid foundation for a transparent, faithful, and deeply connected relationship.

Shared Interests and Intellectual Connection:

- **A meeting of minds**: Age-gap relationships often blossom around shared passions, be it literature, art, travel, or philosophy. These shared interests become fertile grounds for deep intellectual and emotional connections.

- **Learning and evolving together**: The beauty of a mixed-age relationship is the blend of youthful curiosity and seasoned knowledge. This dynamic encourages both partners to explore new interests and share insights, enriching their shared journey.

- **Endless conversations**: A robust intellectual connection ensures that the relationship never lacks stimulating conversations. From debating world events to sharing personal stories, the dialogue is always alive, vibrant, and meaningful.

Financial Stability and Security:

- **A comforting assurance**: Financial stability, often associated with older individuals due to their years in the workforce, provides a sense of security. This stability can offer a comforting assurance in a world filled with uncertainties.

- **Shared financial goals**: A mature partner often brings clarity to financial goals, be it investments, savings, or future planning. This clarity can help in charting a shared financial journey, fostering mutual growth.

- **Lesser financial conflicts**: Studies have often shown that financial disagreements can strain relationships. The financial stability and experience in managing money that an older partner brings can lead to a more harmonious relationship, with fewer conflicts over monetary matters.

Physical attraction might be the initial pull, but the pillars that sustain age-gap relationships are deep, emotional, intellectual, and, at times, practical. It's a world where hearts and minds meet, where shared dreams are woven, and where the assurance of stability provides the comforting warmth in life's cold spells. This profound connection, rooted in mutual respect and shared journeys, truly sets age-gap romances apart.

***

Common Misconceptions

Age-gap relationships, while enchanting and profound, have not been immune to societal scrutiny. Over the years, numerous misconceptions have clouded the understanding of such relationships. They've been romanticized, vilified, misunderstood, and judged. But, to truly appreciate the beauty of these connections, it's crucial to sift fact from fiction. In this chapter, we'll dismantle some widespread myths and set the record straight.

Debunking Stereotypes:

- **Gold diggers and sugar daddies**: One of the most common stereotypes is that younger partners are only in it for the money, while older partners are seeking physical attraction. While financial security or physical appeal might play a role in some relationships, it's reductionist to assume that's all there is to age-gap romances.

- **Lack of common interests**: Many believe that age-gap couples cannot possibly share common interests due to their age difference. However, interests are not solely a product of age. Many couples bond over shared passions, be it music, literature, travel, or countless other pursuits.

- **Short-lived passion**: A prevalent notion is that age-gap relationships are fleeting and don't last. However, like any relationship, the longevity depends on mutual respect, understanding, and effort—not age.

The Difference Between Preference and Fetish:

- **Understanding preference**: Everyone has preferences in relationships, be it based on personality, interests, or age. A preference for older partners is simply an inclination towards the qualities and experiences they bring to the relationship.

- **Defining fetish**: Fetishizing is an unhealthy obsession based solely on a particular aspect, like age. It's superficial and often devoid of deeper emotional connection. While some might have an age fetish, it's crucial to distinguish between genuine age-gap relationships and those rooted in mere fetish.

- **Navigating the thin line**: It's essential to introspect and understand one's motivations. A relationship based on mutual respect and genuine connection, irrespective of age preference, stands on solid ground, while one built on fetish is likely to crumble.

Challenging Societal Judgments:

- **Under the microscope**: Age-gap couples often find themselves under societal scrutiny. While some face benign curiosity, others confront disapproval or judgment. It's crucial to recognize that every relationship is unique, and blanket judgments are both unjust and unfounded.

- **Rising above**: Rather than seeking external validation, couples should focus on their mutual happiness and understanding. Addressing misconceptions through open conversations can also pave the way for broader societal acceptance.

- **Building a support system**: Surrounding oneself with understanding friends and family can provide a buffer against societal judgments. This support system can offer both solace and strength in navigating the challenges.

Misconceptions about age-gap relationships, like mist, often cloud the beautiful landscape of genuine connections. But by challenging these myths and understanding the nuances, we can appreciate the depth and authenticity of such romances. It's not about the years that separate two individuals but the shared moments, dreams, and bonds that bring them together.

***

Gaining Personal Clarity

Age-gap romances, like any profound journey, require introspection. Before plunging into the world of dating older men, it's essential to gain clarity about one's motives, desires, and feelings. Are you genuinely drawn to the maturity and wisdom of an older partner, or is it a mere escapade? Is it a deep-seated preference or a fleeting intrigue kindled by societal narratives? Let's navigate these introspective waters and unearth the true motivations behind seeking an age-gap romance.

Understanding Your Motives:

- **Self-reflection**: The first step towards gaining clarity is self-reflection. It's vital to ask oneself what draws you towards dating older men. Is it their life experience, emotional stability, or simply a pattern you've noticed in your dating history?

- **Past relationship patterns**: Looking back at previous relationships can offer insights. If you've consistently been drawn to older partners, understanding the why can provide clarity on your preferences.

- **Deep-seated desires vs. fleeting fascinations**: It's crucial to discern if your inclination is a deep-rooted desire or a fleeting fascination. While both are valid, recognizing the difference can guide your relationship journey more authentically.

Recognizing Genuine Interest vs. Societal Pressure:

- **Media influence**: Movies, TV shows, and literature often romanticize age-gap relationships. While these narratives can be alluring, it's vital to understand if they influence your preferences or if your desires stem from genuine personal feelings.

- **Peer dynamics**: Sometimes, the circle we keep or the stories we hear from friends can influence our choices. Are your interests in dating older men genuine, or is it a product of wanting to fit into certain peer dynamics?

- **Inner voice vs. external chatter**: Listening to your inner voice amidst the cacophony of societal opinions can be challenging but crucial. It's essential to ensure that your interest is genuinely yours and not an echo of external pressures.

Being Genuine in Your Pursuits:

- **Honesty with oneself**: As you navigate the world of age-gap romances, continually check in with yourself. Ensure that you're being honest with your feelings and not merely going along with a trend.

- **Honesty with potential partners**: It's equally vital to be transparent with older partners you're dating. If you're in it for the experience, adventure, or genuine long-term commitment, communicating your intentions can build trust and understanding.

- **Seeking meaningful connections**: Beyond age, seek connections rooted in shared interests, mutual respect, and emotional depth. This genuine pursuit will ensure that your age-gap romance is fulfilling and meaningful.

Personal clarity is the compass that guides us in the vast ocean of relationships. Especially in age-gap romances, where societal narratives and personal feelings intertwine, this compass becomes indispensable. By understanding our motives, recognizing genuine interests, and being genuine in our pursuits, we can navigate this journey authentically, finding connections that resonate deeply with our souls.

***

Age as Just a Number

The adage "Age is just a number" has been reiterated time and again, but its depth is often overlooked. In relationships, especially age-gap romances, it's imperative to understand that age, in its chronological sense, can sometimes be an arbitrary measure. Two people might be years apart, yet they could share profound connections, understanding, and maturity that transcend their birth years. On the flip side, same-age couples might find mismatches in emotional depth or life perspectives. Let's delve into the nuanced dance between age, maturity, and life experience in relationships.

The Arbitrary Nature of Chronological Age:

- **Beyond birthdays**: While our birth year gives a numerical age, it often doesn't encapsulate our emotional age, maturity, or life experience. A younger individual could possess wisdom beyond their years, while an older person might have a youthful spirit.

- **Cultural contexts**: Different cultures have varied views on age and maturity. In some societies, turning a certain age might be a rite of passage, while in others, life experiences dictate maturity more than age.

- **The fluidity of age perceptions**: How we perceive age and its importance in relationships can change over time. Personal growth, experiences, and changing priorities can make age considerations more fluid than rigid.

Recognizing Maturity Mismatches in Same-Age Relationships:

- **Emotional maturity**: Being of the same age doesn't guarantee emotional compatibility. One partner might be ready for commitment, deep conversations, or future planning, while the other might not.

- **Life goals and priorities**: Same-age partners can have vastly different life goals or priorities. One might prioritize career growth, while the other values travel or personal exploration. Recognizing these mismatches is crucial for relationship harmony.

- **Communication styles**: Maturity also reflects in communication. While both partners might be of the same age, one might possess the maturity to communicate effectively, handle conflicts, or express emotions better than the other.

Age vs. Life Experience: A Balancing Act:

- **Shared journeys**: Age-gap relationships thrive when partners share life experiences or journeys, regardless of their age difference. A shared experience, like traveling, facing similar challenges, or mutual growth pursuits, can form strong bonds.

- **Valuing life lessons**: Every individual, young or old, brings unique life lessons to a relationship. In age-gap romances, it's essential to value these insights, be it the youthful zest of the younger partner or the seasoned wisdom of the older one.

- **Navigating life stages**: Different age stages come with distinct challenges and priorities. Understanding and supporting each other through these life stages, be it career shifts, personal growth, or health challenges, is crucial in age-gap relationships.

In the realm of love and connection, age often blurs into the background. What truly stands out are shared moments, mutual respect, understanding, and the profound connections that two souls forge. Whether it's an age-gap romance or a same-age relationship, it's the depth of connection that truly matters, making age, in its mere numerical sense, just a number.

Chapter Three

Communication is Key

"The single biggest problem in communication is the illusion that it has taken place." – George Bernard Shaw

In any relationship, communication acts as the backbone, the glue that binds two individuals together. In age-gap romances, the importance of communication is accentuated further. With the potential of differences in generational perspectives, life experiences, and stages in personal journeys, effective communication becomes paramount. It's the bridge that helps traverse the age difference, ensuring mutual understanding, trust, and harmony. This chapter will guide you through the intricacies of effective communication in age-gap relationships, emphasizing the nuances and techniques specific to such romances.

Understanding Generational Differences:

- **The cultural gap**: Different generations grow up with varying cultural references, be it music, movies, or societal events.

Recognizing these differences and sharing them can become a delightful learning experience rather than a point of conflict.

- **Values and beliefs**: Over time, societal values and beliefs evolve. It's essential to understand and respect where each partner is coming from, ensuring that generational differences in values don't become points of contention.

- **Technological evolution**: The rapid advancement of technology means different generations might have varied comfort levels with technology. Being patient and teaching (or learning) can be an enriching experience.

Active Listening: More than Hearing:

- **The art of presence**: Active listening is more than just hearing words. It's about being present, understanding the emotions, and grasping the unsaid between the lines.

- **Validating feelings**: In age-gap relationships, where life experiences might differ, validating your partner's feelings and experiences becomes crucial. It's about acknowledging their perspective, even if you don't necessarily agree.

- **Seeking clarity**: Instead of making assumptions, always seek clarity. If something your older (or younger) partner says is unclear or comes from a generational reference you don't understand, ask. It prevents miscommunications and deepens understanding.

Expressing with Authenticity:

- **Honesty is the best policy**: Especially in age-gap relationships, being genuine about your feelings, concerns, or doubts is crucial. It fosters trust and ensures both partners are on the same page.

- **Balancing emotions**: Emotional expressions are vital, but balance is key. It's essential to express emotions without being overly reactive, especially when discussing sensitive topics related to age or life experiences.

- **Non-verbal cues**: Communication isn't just verbal. Understanding and being aware of non-verbal cues, be it body language, facial expressions, or tone, can provide deeper insights into your partner's feelings.

Navigating Difficult Conversations:

- **Choosing the right time**: Timing is everything. If there's a challenging topic to discuss, choose a time when both you and your partner are relaxed and open to conversation.

- **Empathy first**: Before diving into the content of the conversation, express empathy. Ensure your partner knows you're coming from a place of love and understanding.

- **Seeking solutions together**: Instead of pointing fingers or laying blame, approach difficult conversations with a problem-solving mindset. Look for solutions together, emphasizing teamwork.

Communication in age-gap relationships is a dance—a harmonious balance between understanding generational differences, actively listening, expressing authentically, and navigating difficult conversations with grace. When done right, it bridges the age-gap, ensuring that the number of years becomes inconsequential compared to the depth of connection. Remember, it's not about who's right or wrong; it's about understanding and being understood.

***

Understanding Generational Differences

One of the beautiful challenges of age-gap relationships is navigating the terrain of generational differences. While love is timeless, the ways in which different generations express themselves, their points of reference, and their comfort with technology can vary significantly. Let's delve deeper into understanding these generational gaps and how they manifest in relationships. By doing so, we can transform potential points of contention into opportunities for growth, understanding, and mutual appreciation.

Digital Natives vs. Digital Immigrants:

- **Born into technology**: Digital natives, typically the younger generation, have grown up in a world where technology is a constant. Their comfort with digital devices, social media, and online communication is inherent.

- **Learning the digital language**: Digital immigrants, often the older generation, have witnessed the birth and evolution of digital technology. While they might not have the intuitive grasp that digital natives possess, their perspective is enriched by experiencing both pre-digital and digital eras.

- **Patience and learning**: In age-gap relationships, it's essential for digital natives to show patience and understanding, perhaps even educating their older partners on tech nuances. Conversely, digital immigrants bring a rich perspective of a world before online immediacy, offering a balanced view of digital technology.

Pop Culture and Reference Gaps:

- **The evolving entertainment landscape**: Different generations have their icons, movies, music, and events. For one, it might be The Beatles and vinyl records; for another, it could be BTS and Spotify playlists.

- **Shared experiences**: One of the joys of age-gap relationships can be sharing these cultural references. Introduce your older partner to the movies, shows, or music that defined your youth and vice versa. It's an enriching walk down memory lane for one and a delightful new discovery for the other.

- **Respecting differences**: There will be moments when references fly over each other's heads. Instead of letting it be a point of contention, laugh it off and take the time to explain.

It becomes another bonding moment.

Different Communication Styles and Preferences:

- **The written word vs. the spoken word**: Older generations might prefer phone calls, handwritten letters, or face-to-face conversations. In contrast, younger ones might be more inclined towards texting, instant messaging, or video calls.

- **Emojis, gifs, and memes**: The digital age has brought with it a plethora of new ways to express emotions. While a digital native might send a gif or meme to express feelings, a digital immigrant might be more verbose.

- **Balancing both worlds**: It's essential to recognize and respect these differences. Maybe set 'phone call dates' or write occasional handwritten notes, and also have fun texting or sending each other memes. It's all about finding a balance that caters to both partners.

Understanding generational differences is not just about acknowledging the gaps but embracing them. It's about creating a tapestry of shared experiences, teaching moments, and mutual respect. When navigated with love and patience, these differences can add depth, richness, and layers to age-gap relationships. After all, love is about understanding, and what better way to understand each other than through the lens of time and generational wisdom?

**

Building Bridges

Building a strong and lasting relationship across a generational divide involves intentionally finding common ground. While acknowledging differences is crucial, seeking shared experiences, leveraging technology, and creating new memories together are just as important. They act as bridges, connecting the worldviews of two distinct generations and reinforcing the love and understanding between them. This section sheds light on how to effectively bridge the age gap, ensuring that the number of years between partners becomes merely a footnote in their shared journey.

Finding Shared Experiences:

- **Shared hobbies and interests**: While there might be a generational gap, interests such as reading, hiking, cooking, or art can be timeless. Finding such mutual hobbies can be a foundation for many shared moments.

- **Events and milestones**: Talking about significant life events, like a historical moment both lived through (albeit at different ages) or personal milestones, can offer mutual insights and a chance to connect on deeper levels.

- **Learn together**: Enroll in a class or workshop together—be it dance, pottery, or a language class. This not only provides a shared experience but also a chance to grow and learn as a unit.

Leveraging Technology to Bridge Gaps:

- **Digital experiences**: Engage in online activities together, like watching a movie through a streaming service, playing an online game, or even exploring a digital museum.

- **Teach and learn**: If one partner is tech-savvy, use it as an opportunity to teach the other. Conversely, the less tech-inclined partner can share experiences or skills from their era.

- **Using apps for connection**: There are numerous apps designed to help couples stay connected, irrespective of age. From shared calendars to apps that help foster intimacy, leverage them to stay in sync.

Creating New Memories Together:

- **Traveling**: Journey to places neither has been before. This ensures that both partners are on equal footing, exploring and creating memories simultaneously.

- **Cultural immersion**: Attend events or places that are alien to both. Be it a genre of music concert, a cultural festival, or a culinary experience—discovering it together makes it special.

- **Documenting the journey**: Create a scrapbook, start a joint journal, or even create a digital album. Documenting shared moments ensures that over time, you have a tangible representation of your journey together, bridging any generational gaps.

Crafting connections in age-gap relationships requires a blend of intention, understanding, and effort. By actively seeking shared experiences, harnessing technology, and creating a treasure trove of shared memories, couples can ensure that age becomes an enriching part of their narrative rather than a barrier. Remember, every bridge built adds another layer of strength to the foundation of the relationship, making it resilient, rich, and rewarding.

***

Navigating Touchy Subjects

Age-gap relationships, while rich and rewarding, come with their unique set of challenges. Among these are touchy subjects that can be difficult to broach. From discussing past relationships to planning a future with the age difference in mind and even addressing societal judgments, these topics require delicacy, understanding, and clear communication. In this section, we will delve into these touchy subjects, offering insights on how to approach them with grace, ensuring that both partners feel heard, understood, and respected.

Discussing Past Relationships and Experiences:

- **Creating a safe space**: Before discussing past relationships, it's vital to create an environment of trust and understanding. Ensure your partner knows that your intent is to share and understand, not judge or compete.

- **Age-related nuances**: Older partners might have a longer history or even past marriages and children. Approach these discussions with empathy, recognizing that every past relationship has shaped the person they are today.

- **Learning and growing**: Use these conversations as opportunities for growth. Understand patterns, lessons learned, and how past experiences can inform your present relationship in a positive manner.

Future Planning with Age in Mind:

- **Health and wellness**: The reality of an older partner potentially facing health challenges before the younger one needs to be addressed. Discuss plans, health routines, and how to support each other in staying fit and healthy.

- **Retirement and financial planning**: An older partner might retire while the younger one is still in the workforce. Discuss financial plans, ensuring that both partners are on the same page regarding savings, expenses, and future aspirations.

- **Legacy and long-term planning**: Broach the topic of wills, inheritance, and long-term plans. It might be a delicate subject, but having clarity ensures both partners feel secure in the relationship's future.

Addressing Societal Judgments and Reactions:

- **Building resilience together**: Society often has opinions, especially regarding unconventional relationships. Discuss potential reactions and build a strategy to support and defend each other.

- **Choosing your circle**: Surround yourselves with supportive friends and family. While it's essential to address societal judgments, it's just as vital to have a trusted circle that understands and supports your relationship.

- **Public vs. private**: Decide together on how public you want to be about your relationship. Whether you choose to share openly or keep things private, ensure it's a mutual decision made with both partners' comfort in mind.

Navigating touchy subjects in age-gap relationships requires a delicate balance of transparency, empathy, and mutual respect. By proactively addressing these topics, couples can fortify their bond, ensuring that no external factor or internal doubt can shake the foundation they've built together. Remember, every successful conversation around these sensitive topics only deepens the trust and understanding in the relationship, making it stronger and more resilient against external pressures.

***

Active Listening and Empathy

In every relationship, communication is the cornerstone. But in age-gap romances, with the inherent challenges they bring, active listening and empathy become not just essential but transformative. They act as the bridge between two worlds, ensuring that every conversation, whether light-hearted or profound, deepens the bond and mutual understanding. Let's delve deeper into the art of truly hearing your partner, empathizing with their experiences, and building a robust emotional connection that withstands the test of time and societal judgment.

The Art of Truly Hearing Your Partner:

- **Beyond the words**: Active listening isn't just about hearing the words but understanding the emotions, intentions, and sentiments behind them. Pay attention to non-verbal cues like body language, tone, and facial expressions.

- **Avoid interrupting**: Even if you feel the urge to respond, let your partner finish their thoughts. This shows respect and allows for a comprehensive understanding of their perspective.

- **Feedback and clarification**: Once your partner finishes speaking, paraphrase what you've understood, ask clarifying questions, and provide feedback. This ensures that miscommunications are minimized.

Stepping into Their Shoes:

- **Understanding generational emotions**: Recognize that

growing up in different eras comes with varied emotional baggage. By understanding these emotional nuances, you can better empathize with your partner's reactions and perspectives.

- **Seeking shared experiences**: Actively seek situations where you can experience your partner's world. This could mean revisiting a place from their past, diving into their favorite book, or engaging in a shared hobby.

- **Validation**: While you might not always agree, validate your partner's feelings. Let them know that their emotions and experiences are valid and that you understand where they're coming from, even if your perspective differs.

Building Emotional Connections:

- **Sharing vulnerabilities**: Create a safe space where both of you can openly share your vulnerabilities, fears, and dreams. This raw openness can forge deep emotional connections.

- **Regular check-ins**: Set aside regular times to check in with each other emotionally. Understand how each one is feeling, and any challenges faced, and celebrate small victories together.

- **Nurturing mutual growth**: Empathy and active listening are the bedrock for personal and mutual growth. Encourage each other in individual pursuits and celebrate each other's successes, knowing that every achievement, big or small, strengthens the relationship's foundation.

Embracing active listening and empathy is akin to nurturing the very soul of an age-gap relationship. By truly hearing your partner and empathetically stepping into their world, you weave a tapestry of understanding, mutual respect, and deep emotional connection. Remember, in the dance of love, it's not the steps that matter but the rhythm of two hearts beating in unison, and nothing attune those heartbeats better than genuine listening and heartfelt empathy.

***

Handling Disagreements

Every relationship, no matter how harmonious, will face disagreements. In age-gap relationships, these conflicts can sometimes be accentuated by generational differences and inherent power dynamics. However, disagreements, when navigated correctly, can be an avenue for growth, deepening understanding, and reinforcing the relationship's foundation. In this section, we'll explore how to wisely choose battles, recognize and manage age-related power dynamics, and employ strategies for a healthy conflict resolution that leaves both partners feeling valued and heard.

Choosing Battles Wisely:

- **Differentiate between major and minor issues**: Understand that not every disagreement needs to escalate into a full-blown argument. Determine what issues are core to the relationship's health and which ones can be let go.

- **Reflection before reaction**: Before diving headlong into a conflict, take a moment to reflect on its root cause. Often, disagreements stem from external stressors or personal insecurities rather than the matter at hand.

- **Emphasize mutual goals**: Focus on what both of you seek in the relationship—love, understanding, and growth. By emphasizing these shared aspirations, many conflicts can be seen in a different light, leading to easier resolutions.

Recognizing Age-Related Power Dynamics:

- **Be aware of the imbalance**: The older partner might, unintentionally, use their age and experience as a leverage point in disagreements. Recognizing this dynamic is the first step in ensuring it doesn't dictate the relationship's narrative.

- **Encourage equality**: Foster a culture where both voices are equal. Whether it's decision-making or conflict resolution, ensure that both partners have an equal say.

- **Open dialogues**: Regularly discuss and address any feelings of imbalance. By keeping the channels of communication open, both partners can work towards a relationship free of unwanted power plays.

Strategies for Healthy Conflict Resolution:

- **Seek understanding, not victory**: Instead of trying to 'win' an argument, focus on understanding your partner's perspective. This shifts the dynamic from confrontation to conversation.

- **Use "I" statements**: Instead of saying "You always..." or "You never...", express how you feel using "I feel..." or "I believe...". This reduces blame and fosters understanding.

- **Take timeouts**: If a disagreement is getting too heated, it's okay to take a break. Step away, reflect, and return to the conversation with a clearer mind and calmer demeanor.

Handling disagreements with grace, understanding, and a focus on mutual growth can turn potential conflicts into opportunities for a deeper connection. By choosing battles wisely, being mindful of power dynamics, and adopting healthy conflict resolution strategies, age-gap couples can ensure that their relationship remains resilient, vibrant, and nurturing, even in the face of challenges. Remember, it's not about avoiding the storm but learning how to dance in the rain together.

Chapter Four

Navigating the Financial Landscape

"Money is only a tool. It will take you wherever you wish, but it will not replace you as the driver." – Ayn Rand

Money, finances, and the intricate dynamics they bring into a relationship are often some of the most challenging areas to navigate, especially in age-gap relationships. The older partner may be in a different phase of their financial journey, perhaps more settled or even nearing retirement, while the younger partner might be in the throes of building their career or dealing with student loans. It's crucial to find harmony in these potentially contrasting financial landscapes to ensure a relationship's longevity and mutual satisfaction. This chapter aims to guide couples through these financial intricacies, offering strategies to build a stable and mutually beneficial fiscal foundation.

1. Understanding Each Other's Financial Philosophies:

- **Financial upbringings**: Delve into each other's financial histories, understanding how past experiences have shaped monetary beliefs and habits.

- **Goals and aspirations**: Discuss short-term and long-term financial goals. Whether it's buying a home, traveling, or investing, ensure both partners are aligned or at least understand each other's aspirations.

- **Budgeting styles**: Understand how each partner views and handles budgets. This can help in creating a mutual budget that respects individual preferences.

2. Addressing the Income Gap:

- **Transparency is key**: If there's a significant income disparity, be transparent about earnings, expenses, and financial obligations. This fosters trust and mitigates potential misunderstandings.

- **Joint vs. separate accounts**: Discuss if you'd like joint accounts, separate accounts, or a combination of both. This can help in managing expenses in a way that feels equitable to both.

- **Contributions, not percentages**: Instead of splitting expenses 50/50, consider contributing based on income or what each partner is comfortable with, ensuring that no one feels overburdened.

3. Planning for the Future:

- **Retirement plans**: Given the age difference, retirement timelines may differ. Discuss plans, savings, and how both partners envision their golden years.

- **Estate planning**: Consider wills, assets, and how you'd like to handle your financial legacy. This can be a sensitive topic but is essential to address.

- **Investments and growth**: Explore investment opportunities together. Whether it's real estate, stocks, or other ventures, ensure both partners are informed and involved.

4. Addressing Debt and Financial Obligations:

- **Full disclosure**: If either partner has significant debt, it's crucial to be open about it, discussing repayment plans and potential impacts on shared financial goals.

- **Support, not rescue**: Be there for each other, offering support in financial challenges, but avoid fostering a rescuer-rescuee dynamic.

- **Financial literacy**: Consider taking financial workshops or consulting with a financial planner together. This can provide tools and insights to handle debts and plan for a secure financial future.

5. Celebrating Financial Milestones:

- **Acknowledge achievements**: Whether it's paying off debt, reaching a savings goal, or making a significant purchase, celebrate these milestones together.

- **Regular financial check-ins**: Set aside time regularly, maybe once a month or quarterly, to review financial goals, discuss challenges, and recalibrate if necessary.

- **Building together**: Always remember that while individual achievements are great, it's the shared financial journey and growth that strengthens the bond in a relationship.

Navigating the financial landscape in an age-gap relationship requires transparency, understanding, and mutual respect. By addressing potential challenges head-on, fostering open communication, and celebrating financial milestones together, couples can create a fiscal harmony that supports and enhances their shared journey of love and partnership. After all, while money might make the world go round, it's love, understanding, and shared aspirations that truly enrich our lives.

***

Understanding Financial Dynamics

The intricate dance of finances in any relationship can be likened to a delicate ballet. Every move, every pivot, holds significance. Especially in age-gap relationships, where the older partner might be more financially stable, it's essential to understand the dynamics that money can introduce. Money can often be intertwined with power, influencing decisions and dynamics in subtle and not-so-subtle ways. Let's delve deeper into understanding these financial dynamics, ensuring that money becomes a tool for mutual growth rather than a source of contention.

The Potential Power Play:

- **Recognizing inherent dynamics**: With financial stability often comes an inherent sense of power. It's crucial for both partners to recognize this, ensuring that financial stability doesn't translate into dictating terms in the relationship.

- **Open dialogues**: Maintaining open channels of communication can help address any feelings of imbalance or power dynamics due to financial disparities.

- **Setting boundaries**: It's essential to establish financial boundaries early on, ensuring that both partners feel comfortable with shared financial decisions and dynamics.

Financial Independence vs. Interdependence:

- **Valuing individual autonomy**: While it's beneficial to have shared financial goals and responsibilities, it's equally vital to ensure that both partners maintain a sense of financial independence. This means having the autonomy to make individual financial decisions without feeling restricted.

- **Creating a shared financial vision**: Interdependence involves creating a mutual financial vision, wherein both partners contribute to and benefit from shared financial goals and responsibilities.

- **Balancing act**: Striking a balance between financial independence and interdependence can be challenging but is key to ensuring a healthy financial relationship. This could mean having separate accounts for personal expenses and a joint account for shared responsibilities.

Older Men and Financial Responsibilities:

- **Historical perspective**: Historically, men, especially older ones, have often been seen as the primary breadwinners and thus held significant financial responsibilities. Understanding this context can shed light on the financial expectations and pressures they might feel.

- **Shared responsibilities**: In modern relationships, it's essential to move away from traditional financial roles and work towards shared financial responsibilities, ensuring that both partners contribute and have a say in financial matters.

- **Open conversations**: Discuss any preconceived notions or expectations related to financial responsibilities. For instance, if the older man feels a need to take on most of the financial responsibilities, it's essential to discuss this, understand the underlying reasons, and ensure that it aligns with the relationship's mutual vision.

Understanding and navigating the financial dynamics in an age-gap relationship requires empathy, transparency, and constant communication. Recognizing potential power plays, fostering both financial independence and interdependence, and challenging traditional notions of financial responsibilities can pave the way for a harmonious and mutually beneficial financial journey. At the end of the day, money is just a tool – it's the shared dreams, goals, and love that truly define the worth of a relationship.

***

Open Discussions on Money Matters

Finances, for many, remain a taboo subject, shrouded in mystery and hesitation. However, in the context of a romantic relationship, especially one marked by an age gap, it becomes imperative to have open and honest conversations about money. It's not merely about the numbers; it's about the values, the dreams, the fears, and the aspirations that those numbers represent. By laying the foundations of transparency and establishing clear boundaries, couples can fortify their bond against the potential financial storms that life may bring. This chapter delves into the importance of, and strategies for, cultivating open discussions on money matters.

Establishing Transparency from the Start:

- **The value of vulnerability**: Being transparent about financial matters requires a certain level of vulnerability. By openly discussing earnings, debts, savings, and financial goals, both partners can foster a deeper understanding and trust.

- **Consistent check-ins**: Regular financial discussions, be they weekly, monthly, or quarterly, can help keep both partners on the same page and address any concerns or changes in financial situations.

- **No judgment zone**: Ensure that these discussions are a safe space, free from judgments or criticisms. It's about understanding and supporting each other, not about pointing fingers.

Discussing Financial Boundaries:

- **The importance of boundaries**: Financial boundaries help in setting clear expectations about spending limits, shared responsibilities, and individual financial autonomy. They act as safeguards, ensuring that both partners feel respected and valued in their financial contributions and decisions.

- **Drafting a financial agreement**: While it may seem formal, drafting a mutual financial agreement can be beneficial. It can outline shared expenses, investment strategies, and other financial responsibilities, ensuring clarity and minimizing potential disputes.

- **Revisiting and revising**: As with all things in life, financial situations and goals can evolve. Regularly revisiting and, if necessary, revising established boundaries can help in staying aligned with changing circumstances and aspirations.

Planning for Financial Emergencies:

- **The inevitability of the unexpected**: Life is unpredictable. Whether it's a sudden job loss, a medical emergency, or an unexpected expense, financial emergencies can arise. Preparing for them is key.

- **Building an emergency fund**: This is a fund explicitly set aside to handle unforeseen expenses. Both partners can contribute to it, deciding on a mutual target amount based on their combined incomes and potential expenses.

- **Insurance and long-term planning**: Apart from an emergency fund, consider investments in health, life, and property insurance. Also, discussing long-term financial strategies can provide an added layer of security against potential financial adversities.

Openness in financial discussions cultivates a relationship's core strength. It's not merely about sharing numbers but about sharing dreams, fears, and hopes. By establishing transparency, setting clear boundaries, and preparing for the unexpected, couples can navigate the often turbulent waters of finances with grace, understanding, and mutual respect. After all, it's not the challenges but how we face them together that truly defines the depth and resilience of a relationship.

***

Building Joint Financial Goals

Money is more than just currency; it's a tangible reflection of shared dreams, aspirations, and values. As a couple, particularly in an age-gap relationship, aligning your financial visions becomes paramount. While both partners may come from different financial backgrounds and have diverse experiences, the act of setting joint goals allows for the harmonization of those differences into a cohesive, shared plan. From dream vacations to retirement plans, this chapter explores the importance of and strategies for building joint financial goals, ensuring a future that both partners can look forward to with excitement and security.

Planning for the Future: Vacations, Properties, Investments:

- **Dreaming together**: Start by visualizing mutual aspirations. Whether it's a dream vacation to the Maldives, buying a cozy cottage by the lakeside, or investing in a promising start-up, laying out these dreams sets the stage for financial planning.

- **Creating a timeline**: Assign tentative timelines to each goal. For instance, if you both aim to buy a property in the next five years, that timeline will guide your saving and investment decisions.

- **Research and strategize**: Once goals and timelines are set, dive into the research. Understand the costs involved, explore potential investment opportunities, and strategize on how best to achieve these goals.

Discussing Retirement Plans:

- **Recognizing the age difference**: In age-gap relationships, retirement can be a unique consideration. One partner may be nearing retirement while the other is in the prime of their career. Understand the implications of this.

- **Syncing retirement visions**: While one might dream of a quiet countryside life, the other might envision globetrotting adventures. Discussing and aligning these visions is key.

- **Financial considerations**: Discuss the financial aspects of retirement, including potential pensions, savings, investments, and any other income sources. Consider the implications of early or late retirement and strategize accordingly.

Setting Mutual Financial Priorities:

- **Needs vs. Wants**: Understand the distinction between what's essential and what's desirable. While a vacation might be a want, setting aside money for an emergency might be a need. Prioritize accordingly.

- **Flexibility is key**: Recognize that financial priorities can change. Regular check-ins allow both partners to reassess and realign their priorities as life evolves.

- **Celebrate milestones**: As you achieve your financial goals, no matter how big or small, take a moment to celebrate. It not only fosters a sense of accomplishment but also strengthens the bond between partners.

Crafting joint financial goals is akin to painting a canvas of the future – filled with colors of dreams, strokes of aspirations, and the nuances of shared values. While the process requires understanding, patience, and compromise, the result is a masterpiece that both partners can cherish. After all, the journey towards a shared future, paved with mutual dreams and goals, is what truly makes a relationship rich in every sense.

***

Maintaining Financial Independence

In the dance of romance, particularly in age-gap relationships, there is a subtle play of interdependence and individuality. While building joint financial goals is crucial, maintaining one's financial independence within the relationship is equally, if not more, important. It's not just about money; it's about self-esteem, empowerment, and autonomy. By nurturing personal financial security and growth, individuals not only safeguard their future but also bring a stronger, more confident self into the relationship. This chapter delves into the significance of, and strategies for, maintaining financial independence while being an integral part of a duo.

The Importance of Personal Financial Security:

- **Empowerment and self-worth**: Personal financial security fosters a sense of empowerment, giving individuals the confidence to make decisions and face challenges head-on.

- **A safety net**: While we hope for the best in relationships, life is unpredictable. Having one's financial security provides a safety net, ensuring stability even in tumultuous times.

- **Enhancing relationship dynamics**: When both partners are financially secure, the relationship dynamics tend to be more balanced, minimizing potential power plays or dependencies.

Strategies for Financial Growth:

- **Diversifying income sources**: Relying on a single income stream can be risky. Exploring side hustles, investments, or other revenue-generating avenues can bolster financial growth.

- **Continuous learning**: The financial world is ever-evolving. Regularly educating oneself on the latest investment strategies, financial tools, or market trends can be beneficial.

- **Seeking expert advice**: Consulting with financial advisors or experts can provide valuable insights, guiding one's financial growth journey.

Setting Personal Financial Boundaries:

- **Clear delineation**: While pooling resources for shared goals is vital, it's equally important to have clear boundaries on personal finances. This could involve separate bank accounts, designated personal savings, or defined spending limits.

- **Open communication**: Regularly discuss personal financial boundaries with your partner. This not only ensures clarity but also builds mutual respect for each other's financial autonomy.

- **Review and adapt**: Just as joint financial goals may evolve, personal financial boundaries might also need revisiting. Adapting these boundaries in light of changing circumstances or aspirations ensures continued financial independence.

Independence and unity are not mutually exclusive. In the tapestry of a relationship, the threads of individuality and togetherness weave together to create a resilient and beautiful fabric. By maintaining financial independence, individuals not only empower themselves but also enrich the relationship with trust, respect, and mutual admiration. After all, two independent individuals choosing to be together, while honoring each other's autonomy, make the strongest and most harmonious duos.

***

Legal and Financial Precautions

Love is a beautiful emotion, but when it comes to age-gap relationships, certain practicalities cannot be overlooked. As with any substantial venture in life, love too requires a solid foundation built on trust, understanding, and preparedness. This is especially true when the relationship entails significant age differences, bringing in unique financial and legal considerations. From prenuptial agreements to planning for the eventualities of life, this chapter underscores the importance of and provides guidance on fortifying the foundation of your relationship with necessary legal and financial precautions.

Prenuptial Agreements and Why They Matter:

- **Protection of assets**: Prenups are not just about distrust or expecting the relationship to fail. It's a pragmatic approach to protect assets that one brings into a marriage, especially crucial in age-gap relationships where one partner may have accumulated substantial wealth.

- **Clarifying financial expectations**: A prenup allows for open dialogue about financial expectations, responsibilities, and any potential alimony or spousal support.

- **Minimizing potential conflicts**: In the unfortunate event of a breakup, having a prenup can streamline the process, reducing potential conflicts and ensuring a fair division.

Wills, Testaments, and Inheritance:

- **Expressing your wishes**: A will ensures that your assets are distributed as per your desires, offering clarity and avoiding potential disputes among heirs.

- **Accounting for age differences**: In age-gap relationships, the older partner might have children from previous relationships or other family members they wish to include in their will. Ensuring that all loved ones are fairly considered is paramount.

- **Seeking legal counsel**: Engage a lawyer to help draft a clear and legally sound will. They can offer guidance on inheritance laws, tax implications, and other nuances.

Financial Planning with Age in Mind:

- **Considering life stages**: Recognize that age-gap couples might be at different life stages, affecting financial goals. One might be focusing on career growth while the other might be nearing retirement.

- **Health and insurance considerations**: As age progresses, health considerations become crucial. Ensure comprehensive health insurance and consider potential long-term care needs.

- **Planning for retirement and beyond:** If one partner is significantly older, consider the financial implications of their potential retirement, the need for assisted living, or other age-related expenses. This requires a comprehensive financial plan that ensures comfort and security in the later years.

While love is the cornerstone of any romantic relationship, legal and financial precautions act as the protective walls, ensuring that the relationship stands strong against unforeseen challenges. It's about acknowledging the realities of life while cherishing the bond of love. With the right precautions in place, couples can move forward with confidence, focusing on building a life filled with memories, knowing that they are well-prepared for both the sun and the rain.

Chapter Five

Bridging Cultural and Social Gaps

"*Culture makes people understand each other better.*" – *Paulo Coelho*

When embarking on age-gap relationships, it's not only the chronological difference that couples navigate. The tapestry of such unions often consists of diverse threads from varied cultural, societal, and historical backgrounds. These distinctions add richness to the relationship but can also present challenges. The beauty lies in understanding, appreciating, and bridging these gaps, turning potential conflicts into avenues for growth and deeper connection. In this chapter, we delve deep into recognizing these cultural and social differences and provide guidance on how to harmoniously weave them into your love story.

Recognizing Differences and Similarities:

- **Generational insights**: Each generation is molded by the events, technologies, and cultural shifts of its time. Recognize the influences that have shaped each partner and appreciate the perspectives they bring.

- **Shared human experiences**: While cultural and social backgrounds might differ, many human emotions and experiences are universal. Find common ground in shared feelings, aspirations, and dreams.

- **Respecting individual histories**: Both partners bring their unique stories, values, and traditions. Celebrate these individual histories as they form the essence of who you both are.

Open Dialogue and Curiosity:

- **Ask, don't assume**: Assumptions can lead to misunderstandings. Approach differences with genuine curiosity, asking questions to truly understand your partner's perspective.

- **Share personal stories**: Bond over memories, experiences, and tales from your respective pasts. This can be a fun and enlightening way to understand each other's worlds.

- **Seek feedback**: Encourage your partner to share their feelings about any cultural or social habits you have, ensuring that both parties feel valued and understood.

Adapting and Integrating:

- **Celebrate traditions**: Embrace each other's cultural and social traditions, be it festivals, foods, or family rituals. Make them a part of your joint narrative.

- **Learning together**: Engage in activities like attending cultural events, reading, or watching documentaries that provide insights into each other's backgrounds.

- **Creating a shared culture**: While cherishing individual cultures, also focus on creating a unique shared culture that embodies elements from both worlds.

Navigating Social Perceptions and Judgments:

- **Building resilience**: Society often has preconceived notions about age-gap relationships. Develop resilience against unwarranted judgments, focusing on the strength of your bond.

- **Finding supportive communities**: Engage with communities or groups that are open-minded and supportive, providing a safe space to share experiences and seek advice.

- **Educating naysayers**: When faced with skepticism or negativity, use it as an opportunity to educate and share the beauty of your relationship.

Seeking External Support:

- **Couple's therapy**: Consider attending couples therapy that focuses on multicultural or age-gap relationships. Therapists can provide tools and strategies to navigate challenges effectively.

- **Mentorship**: Seek mentorship from other age-gap couples who have successfully navigated similar challenges. Their insights and advice can be invaluable.

- **Continuous learning**: The journey of understanding cultural and social gaps is ongoing. Remain open to learning, evolving, and growing together as a unit.

In a world that is increasingly interconnected, age-gap relationships are a testament to the power of love that transcends boundaries. By recognizing, understanding, and embracing cultural and social differences, couples can create a union that is rich in diversity and united in love. Remember, it's the myriad of colors that make a rainbow beautiful; similarly, it's the blend of two diverse worlds that adds depth, flavor, and beauty to age-gap relationships.

***

Generational Culture Shock

Every generation is a distinct tapestry woven with the threads of its defining moments, be it world events, technological advancements, or cultural revolutions. These formative experiences create unique societal norms, values, and cultural touchstones that resonate deeply with individuals of that era. When two people from different generations come together in a romantic relationship, these differences can sometimes lead to a "culture shock." This section will explore the intricacies of such generational distinctions and offer insights into navigating them harmoniously.

Shifts in Societal Norms and Values:

- **Understanding the influences**: Societal values don't change in a vacuum. Events like wars, social movements, and technological disruptions heavily influence generational perspectives. Recognize the major events that shaped each partner's era to understand the foundation of their values.

- **Embracing evolution**: Realize that societal norms evolve. What was considered taboo or unconventional in one generation might be mainstream in another. Approach these shifts with an open mind.

- **Finding common values**: Despite changes, core human values like love, respect, and understanding often remain consistent. Focus on these shared principles to find common ground.

Music, Films, and Entertainment Across Generations:

- **Taking a walk down memory lane**: Share your favorite movies, songs, and shows from your generation. It's not just about entertainment but also about understanding the cultural nuances, themes, and sentiments of the time.

- **Exploring together**: Designate "retro nights" where you indulge in classics from each other's era or "contemporary nights" to explore current entertainment. It's a fun way to bond and understand generational tastes.

- **Appreciating the evolution**: Art reflects life. Notice the shifts in genres, storytelling styles, or musical compositions over the years. Appreciate the richness that each era brings to the world of entertainment.

Navigating Political and Social Opinions:

- **Safe spaces for discussion**: Differences in political and social opinions can be sensitive. Ensure discussions are approached as dialogues, not debates. Aim to understand, not to convince.

- **Recognizing generational influences**: Many political and social opinions are shaped by the events of one's formative years. Acknowledge this context when discussing differing views.

- **Agreeing to disagree**: It's okay to have different opinions. The key is respect. Ensure that differing views don't lead to personal judgments or assumptions.

Age-gap relationships can be a journey through time, allowing partners to experience the best of different eras. While generational culture shock is natural, it can also be an enriching experience, filled with discoveries, learning, and deepening of the bond. As you navigate these differences, remember that it's not about changing for each other but growing with each other.

***

Building Shared Cultural Experiences

Cultural touchstones act as anchors, connecting us to our roots and giving a sense of belonging and identity. When two individuals from different generations come together, they bring with them a wealth of cultural experiences, memories, and references. Merging these distinct worlds can be a delightful journey, one that enriches the relationship and creates a unique shared narrative. This section dives into the art of building shared cultural experiences that celebrate both the diversity and unity of age-gap relationships.

Introducing Each Other to Cultural Touchstones:

- **Share stories**: The stories we grow up with, be it folk tales, family anecdotes, or historical events, offer a window into our cultural psyche. Take turns to narrate stories that were significant to your generation.

- **Engage in cultural activities**: Attend events, festivals, or places that hold cultural significance for each partner. It could be a rock concert from one's youth or a modern art exhibition that resonates with the other.

- **Culinary journeys**: Food is a powerful cultural ambassador. Introduce each other to dishes, recipes, or cuisines that have a special place in your heart.

Creating a Shared Cultural Lexicon:

- **Developing 'our' language**: Every culture has phrases, idioms, or slang that are deeply rooted in its zeitgeist. Share these with each other and create a playful lexicon that's unique to your relationship.

- **Building a shared playlist**: Music transcends age. Curate a playlist that features favorites from both eras, creating a harmonious blend of old classics and new hits.

- **Shared experiences**: Engage in activities or hobbies that neither has experienced before. This way, you're not just sharing but creating new cultural touchstones together.

Respecting and Valuing Differences:

- **Avoiding stereotypes**: It's easy to resort to generational clichés. Be mindful and avoid making sweeping generalizations about each other's cultures.

- **Embracing the learning curve**: Approach differences with curiosity, not judgment. Recognize that every cultural aspect, no matter how unfamiliar, has its value and significance.

- **Honoring boundaries**: While sharing is beautiful, it's also essential to recognize and respect boundaries. Some cultural rituals or memories might be deeply personal. Understand and respect if your partner wishes to keep certain things private.

Building shared cultural experiences is like crafting a mosaic – each piece, with its unique shape, color, and texture, contributes to the masterpiece. In age-gap relationships, these shared experiences not only strengthen the bond but also create a legacy that's a beautiful blend of both worlds. Embrace the journey with an open heart, a curious mind, and a spirit of adventure.

***

Handling External Judgments

When two souls connect deeply, age becomes a mere number. However, the world outside the relationship might not always see it with the same clarity. External judgments, stigmas, and criticisms can cast a shadow on the most genuine of relationships. But with the right mindset and strategies, couples can navigate these challenges and thrive against the odds. This section offers guidance on facing the world with confidence and grace, holding each other's hand.

Dealing with Societal Stigmas:

- **Understanding the root**: Societal judgments often stem

from deep-rooted stereotypes and misconceptions. Recognizing these biases can help couples navigate them with empathy and patience.

- **Choosing your circle**: Surround yourself with open-minded individuals who value love over societal conventions. This supportive environment can act as a shield against unwarranted criticism.

- **Educating when necessary**: Engage in constructive dialogues to dispel myths around age-gap relationships. Remember, it's not about convincing but sharing your perspective.

Addressing Friends' and Family's Concerns:

- **Open communication**: Initiate conversations with loved ones to understand their concerns. Listening can often be the first step to acceptance.

- **Introducing gradually**: If you anticipate resistance, introduce your partner in informal, low-pressure settings to give your friends and family time to adjust.

- **Seeking counseling**: Family therapy or counseling sessions can be a platform for airing concerns and bridging gaps, especially if resistance persists.

Building Resilience Against Criticism:

- **Internal validation**: Seek validation from within the relationship rather than external sources. Reaffirming your love and commitment to each other can help build resilience against external opinions.

- **Establishing boundaries**: Decide early on which topics are open for discussion and which are off-limits. Setting clear boundaries can prevent unsolicited advice or criticism.

- **Focusing on the positive**: Every relationship has its challenges and joys. Highlight and celebrate the unique advantages of your age-gap relationship to overshadow the criticisms.

Facing external judgments can be challenging, but it's essential to remember that the heart of the relationship lies in the bond shared by the couple. By standing united, building resilience, and navigating challenges with love and understanding, age-gap couples can create a haven that's impervious to the storms of societal opinions. After all, true love, understanding, and commitment are universal languages that defy age and time.

***

Embracing Shared Social Activities

Sharing life together in an age-gap relationship goes beyond just co-existing; it's about actively participating in each other's worlds. Social activities are the tapestry upon which many relationships are built and strengthened. When couples from different generations come together, there is a vast expanse of experiences to share and new memories to create. This section provides a roadmap for couples to embrace shared activities and create a rich, interwoven social life that celebrates both their individualities and shared interests.

Finding Common Hobbies and Pastimes:

- **Exploration sessions**: Dedicate time to trying out different activities together. Be it dancing, painting, hiking, or reading – discover passions you both resonate with.

- **Blending old and new**: Each partner can introduce the other to their favorite hobbies. For instance, a love for vintage vinyl records might merge with a passion for modern digital playlists.

- **Enroll in classes**: Joining classes or workshops can be a fun way to explore shared interests and learn something new together, from cooking to photography.

Introducing Each Other to Social Circles:

- **Host gatherings**: Organize get-togethers where friends and family from both sides can mingle. This can be a relaxed way to integrate your social worlds.

- **Participate in group activities**: Engage in group activities like group trips, game nights, or community events. These shared experiences can help strengthen bonds and ease introductions.

- **Respect comfort zones**: Remember that it might take time for everyone to adjust. Be patient and understanding, giving each person the space they need.

Navigating Social Events with Age Differences:

- **Pre-event communication**: Discuss any potential challenges or sensitivities that might arise at a particular event due to the age difference and strategize how to handle them.

- **Dress the part**: While it's crucial to be oneself, dressing appropriately for an event can help both partners feel confident and mitigate potential age-related attention.

- **Stay united**: Attending social events as a team, and supporting each other, can help navigate any challenges or awkward situations that arise.

When two people, irrespective of their age difference, share activities and socialize together, they're doing more than just passing the time. They're building a shared narrative, one where their worlds intermingle, enriching each other's lives. The key is to approach every activity with an open mind, a willing heart, and a sense of adventure, ensuring that every moment spent together strengthens the bonds of love and understanding.

***

The Power of Compromise

Every relationship, regardless of the age difference, requires compromise. It's the dance of give-and-take, a harmonization of differences that creates a symphony of mutual respect and understanding. In age-gap relationships, where life experiences and generational cultures might differ, the power of compromise becomes even more pronounced. This section offers insights into the delicate art of compromise, allowing couples to flourish amidst their differences and craft a love story that's both rich and resilient.

Balancing Individual and Shared Interests:

- **Creating a shared calendar**: Designate days or moments dedicated to shared activities, while also ensuring there's time for individual pursuits. This balance keeps the relationship fresh and allows personal growth.

- **Supporting solo adventures**: Encourage each other to pursue individual interests, understanding that personal growth contributes to the health of the relationship.

- **Celebrating commonalities**: Actively seek and celebrate shared interests, ensuring they become integral parts of your relationship tapestry.

Respecting Each Other's Comfort Zones:

- **Open dialogues**: Consistent communication is key. Discuss boundaries openly, ensuring each partner feels heard and understood.

- **Prioritizing emotional safety**: Make sure both partners feel emotionally safe when venturing outside their comfort zones, ensuring that any exploration is consensual and enjoyable.

- **Gradual expansion**: Instead of drastic changes, consider gradual shifts that help both partners expand their comfort zones over time.

Finding Joy in Discovery and Exploration:

- **Adventure days**: Dedicate days where you both try something entirely new, be it a cuisine, an activity, or a travel destination. The novelty can reinvigorate the relationship.

- **Documenting the journey**: Create a journal or scrapbook that captures your shared adventures, fostering a sense of shared history.

- **Cherishing the learning curve**: Recognize that every new exploration, even if it doesn't become a favorite, adds a layer to the relationship's story. Celebrate the journey, irrespective of the destination.

In the dance of love, compromise is the rhythm that guides every step. It's not about sacrificing or losing oneself but about co-creating a shared journey that honors both individuals. By understanding the power of compromise, couples can craft a love story that resonates with mutual respect, joy, and a celebration of shared moments. As they weave their narrative together, they'll find that their differences, when harmonized, create a melody that's unique, enduring, and profoundly beautiful.

Chapter Six

Planning for the Future

"*The best way to predict the future is to create it.*" – *Peter Drucker*

When two hearts come together, especially in an age-gap relationship, the journey forward becomes an intricate blend of dreams, aspirations, and practical realities. The future, with its myriad possibilities, requires careful planning and nurturing. Whether it's discussing life goals, retirement, or family dynamics, each conversation becomes an essential stepping stone. This chapter delves deep into the art and science of future planning in age-gap relationships, offering a roadmap for couples to design a future that's as radiant as their love.

1. Setting Mutual Goals:

- **Dreaming together**: Organize sessions where you both discuss and visualize your shared future, ensuring your dreams align.

- **Balancing aspirations**: While it's essential to dream big, it's equally crucial to set achievable and realistic milestones.

- **Periodic check-ins**: Schedule regular conversations to assess the progress of your mutual goals, making adjustments as life evolves.

2. Discussing Family Dynamics:

- **Blended families**: Navigate the complexities of blending families, understanding the needs of children or family members from previous relationships.

- **Introducing family**: Develop strategies for introducing each other to extended families, ensuring smooth integration.

- **Discussing future family plans**: If relevant, explore the possibilities of expanding your family, be it through adoption, childbirth, or other means.

3. Retirement Planning:

- **Age-related considerations**: Given the age difference, discuss individual retirement timelines and what that means for the relationship.

- **Financial preparedness**: Ensure you're both aligned on retirement savings, investments, and other financial planning aspects.

- **Exploring retirement activities**: Discuss how you'd like to spend your retirement years, from travel to hobbies or even starting new ventures together.

4. Health and Wellness Conversations:

- **Age-related health discussions**: Talk about potential health issues related to age and how you both plan to navigate them.

- **Wellness routines**: Design shared health and wellness routines, from exercises to diets, ensuring you both stay fit and happy.

- **Emergency preparedness**: Ensure that both partners are informed and prepared for any unforeseen health emergencies.

5. Legal Considerations:

- **Wills and estate planning**: Discuss and finalize aspects related to wills, ensuring clarity on property distribution, assets, and other legacy concerns.

- **Power of attorney**: Determine who would have the power of attorney in case of emergencies, ensuring that decisions can be made swiftly if required.

- **Life insurance and other policies**: Review life insurance policies and other related instruments to ensure that both partners are adequately covered and beneficiaries are clear.

While the romance of a relationship is its most celebrated aspect, the practicalities of future planning are its backbone. In an age-gap relationship, where life's stages might not always align perfectly, open dialogue and mutual respect become paramount. By charting a course together, couples not only fortify their bond but also create a shared narrative that's rooted in love, trust, and mutual growth. The journey ahead might have its twists and turns, but with careful planning and unwavering commitment, it promises to be an adventure like no other.

***

Discussing Long-term Commitments

Every relationship, at its core, is a journey towards a shared future. Age-gap relationships, with their unique dynamics, often have a distinct set of considerations when planning for the long term. From deciding to move in together, to contemplating marriage, or discussing the possibility of children, each step is crucial. This section delves deep into these essential topics, guiding couples through the intricacies of making long-term commitments and building a life together.

Marriage and its Implications:

- **Understanding legalities**: Age-gap couples, especially with significant differences, might face unique legal considerations when tying the knot. It's essential to be informed and prepared.

- **Pre-marital counseling**: Engaging in counseling sessions can provide valuable insights into potential challenges and equip couples with strategies to overcome them.

- **Discussing ceremonies and traditions**: Integrate elements from both partners' cultural and generational backgrounds to craft a wedding ceremony that reflects the essence of their bond.

Moving in Together: Pros and Cons:

- **Trial period**: Consider living together for a set period before making a permanent decision. This "test drive" can provide insights into compatibility and daily living dynamics.

- **Discussing logistics**: Dive deep into the details— from whose place to move into, to merging belongings and setting up shared spaces.

- **Setting boundaries**: As with any cohabitation, it's vital to discuss and establish personal boundaries to maintain harmony and personal space.

Discussing Potential Children and Blended Families:

- **Open conversations about desires**: It's crucial to be transparent about the desire for children. Does one partner want them, while the other doesn't? Are both on the same page?

These discussions can shape the relationship's future.

- **Navigating blended families**: If one or both partners have children from previous relationships, it's essential to discuss the dynamics of blending these families— integration, relationships, and potential challenges.

- **Seeking external advice**: Consider engaging in family counseling, especially when discussing potential children or navigating blended families. Professional guidance can offer valuable perspectives and solutions.

Envisioning and planning a shared future is an intimate process, filled with excitement, anticipation, and inevitable challenges. By approaching these discussions with honesty, openness, and a commitment to understanding, age-gap couples can lay the foundation for a strong, enduring relationship that thrives in the face of any adversity. Remember, it's not just about charting the course; it's about enjoying the journey, hand in hand.

***

Navigating Health Challenges

Love, in its most profound form, is not just about celebrating the highs but also standing steadfast during the lows. Health challenges, especially in age-gap relationships, can emerge as a focal point of concern. While the younger partner might be in the prime of their health, the older partner might be approaching or already at an age where health challenges become more frequent. This section delves into the delicate and essential topic of health, providing a guide on how couples can navigate these challenges with grace, understanding, and unwavering support.

The Reality of Age and Health:

- **Understanding physiological changes**: With age, certain health issues become more prevalent. Couples should educate themselves on potential health concerns linked to age.

- **Regular check-ups**: For the older partner, routine medical check-ups can help in the early detection and management of health issues. The younger partner should also prioritize health, fostering a mutual culture of well-being.

- **Lifestyle adaptations**: Adopting a healthy lifestyle, including diet and exercise, can play a pivotal role in mitigating age-related health challenges.

Supporting Each Other During Health Crises:

- **Being present**: Sometimes, the best support is merely being there— attending doctor's appointments, holding hands during treatments, or just listening.

- **Seeking external support**: Engage in support groups or counseling that cater specifically to couples navigating health challenges.

- **Fostering resilience**: Develop strategies as a couple to cope with health challenges, focusing on emotional well-being and mental strength.

Discussions about Caregiving and Support:

- **Defining roles and boundaries**: Be clear about what kind of support each partner is willing and able to provide. This includes both physical caregiving and emotional support.

- **Exploring external caregiving options**: Understand that there might be situations where professional caregiving becomes necessary. Be open to discussing these possibilities.

- **Legal and financial preparations**: Discussing potential health challenges should also involve planning for medical emergencies, understanding health insurance, and ensuring legal documents like medical power of attorney are in place.

Facing health challenges can be one of the most testing times in a relationship. However, these challenges can also strengthen bonds, forging connections deeper and more profound than ever before. For age-gap couples, the journey might have its unique hurdles, but with love, understanding, and mutual respect, they can traverse any challenge, emerging stronger and more united than ever.

***

Setting Mutual Goals

Relationships thrive not just on love and understanding but also on shared aspirations and mutual goals. Age-gap couples often bring different perspectives from their respective life stages. However, the beauty lies in weaving these unique threads into a shared tapestry of dreams and aspirations. This section offers a roadmap to help couples set and achieve mutual goals, ensuring that their paths, though distinct, converge in harmony and shared purpose.

Career Aspirations and Retirement:

- **Synchronous planning**: While one partner might be nearing the pinnacle of their career or contemplating retirement, the other might be ascending the career ladder. It's vital to understand and support each other's career trajectories and decisions.

- **Retirement readiness**: Discuss timelines, expectations, and plans for retirement. This could involve a shift in lifestyle, location, or daily routines.

- **Financial preparation**: Align financial plans with career and retirement aspirations, ensuring that both partners are secure and the future is safeguarded.

Travel and Shared Experiences:

- **Bucket list creation**: Make a joint list of places to visit, experiences to seek, and dreams to chase. This shared bucket list becomes a roadmap of adventures waiting to be explored together.

- **Cultural immersion**: Use travel as an opportunity to introduce each other to different facets of your generational experiences. Visit places that hold special significance to each partner.

- **Documenting memories**: Chronicle your journeys, both metaphorical and literal. This could be in the form of journals, blogs, or photo albums, ensuring that memories are preserved.

Building a Legacy Together:

- **Defining a 'legacy'**: Understand what 'legacy' means to each partner. Is it about family, contributions to society, a business venture, or perhaps something more intangible?

- **Collaborative projects**: Engage in projects or ventures as a couple. It could be as simple as a community initiative or as complex as a business endeavor.

- **Passing on wisdom**: Consider ways to pass on knowledge, experiences, and wisdom to younger generations or the community. This could be through mentorship programs, writing, or community teaching.

While the chapters of life each partner has already written might be distinct, the future holds blank pages waiting to be penned together. By setting mutual goals and walking hand in hand towards shared aspirations, age-gap couples can create a compelling narrative of love, unity, and shared purpose, proving that love knows no bounds, not even time.

***

Handling Loss and Grief

Loss and grief are inevitable facets of the human experience. For age-gap couples, the reality of these challenges can often present itself more acutely, given the generational difference. The journey through grief is deeply personal, yet it's also a journey that couples can navigate together, finding strength in each other's support. This section delves into the myriad emotions and challenges associated with loss, providing a guiding light for couples as they wade through the tumultuous waters of grief.

Facing the Reality of Mortality:

- **Open conversations**: Discuss the inevitable nature of life and death, addressing fears, expectations, and wishes. This can pave the way for deeper understanding and shared coping mechanisms.

- **Preparation**: While it's uncomfortable, it's essential to discuss end-of-life wishes, funeral arrangements, and related topics to ensure that both partners' desires are respected.

- **Celebrating life**: Focus on making the most of the present, cherishing each moment together, and creating lasting memories.

Supporting Each Other During Times of Loss:

- **Being present**: The mere act of being there, offering a shoulder to cry on or a listening ear, can be immensely comforting during times of grief.

- **Seeking external support**: Consider counseling, grief support groups, or therapy to navigate the complexities of loss. Sometimes, an external perspective can provide clarity and healing.

- **Remembering together**: Share stories, memories, and experiences of the loved one lost, ensuring that their legacy lives on through shared recollections.

Ensuring Emotional Well-being for Both:

- **Self-care**: While it's crucial to support each other, individual self-care is equally vital. Engage in activities that bring solace and healing.

- **Balancing emotions**: Recognize that grief doesn't have a set timeline. Each partner might cope differently, and it's essential to respect and understand those differences.

- **Building resilience**: Develop coping strategies, rituals, or traditions to commemorate the loved ones lost and find strength in shared experiences.

Navigating the realms of loss and grief can be daunting. Yet, it's during these challenging times that the strength of a relationship shines brightest. For age-gap couples, the journey might be dotted with unique hurdles, but with understanding, patience, and mutual support, they can traverse this challenging path, emerging as pillars of strength for each other. Love, in its truest form, transcends the boundaries of life and death, proving that true connections are indeed eternal.

***

Reassessing and Adapting Goals

As the sands of time flow, so do our desires, aspirations, and circumstances. Just like a river carving its way through landscapes, a relationship too needs to meander through life's changing terrains. Age-gap couples, given the inherent differences in life stages, might often find their goals evolving at a different pace. Embracing these changes, reassessing mutual aspirations, and adapting to the shifting tides can fortify the bond and ensure a relationship that's dynamic, resilient, and ever-evolving. This section serves as a compass for couples navigating these transformations, ensuring their journey remains vibrant and fulfilling.

Periodic Check-ins on Relationship Health:

- **Scheduled reflections**: Set aside dedicated times, be it monthly or annually, for candid discussions about the relationship's state, ensuring both partners feel heard and valued.

- **Feedback loops**: Create a safe space for open feedback, where concerns, joys, and grievances can be aired without judgment.

- **Growth markers**: Identify key milestones or markers that indicate the relationship's health and growth, celebrating successes and addressing areas of concern.

Addressing Changing Aspirations and Desires:

- **Vision boards**: Regularly update joint vision boards, visually capturing evolving dreams, desires, and aspirations.

- **Shared bucket lists**: As dreams are realized or changed, keep updating a shared list of experiences and adventures both partners wish to embark on.

- **Open-mindedness**: Recognize that change is a constant. Being open to adapting and modifying life goals ensures both partners remain aligned in their journey.

Keeping the Spark Alive Amidst Challenges:

- **Date nights**: Regularly carve out time for just the two of you, revisiting the early days of courtship and rekindling the flames of passion.

- **Surprises**: Infuse the relationship with unexpected gestures, gifts, or experiences, keeping the element of surprise and delight alive.

- **Learning together**: Engage in new activities, classes, or hobbies as a couple. This shared learning not only brings freshness but also strengthens the bond.

Life, in all its unpredictability, brings a melange of experiences. For age-gap couples, this dynamism can be both a challenge and an opportunity. By regularly reassessing and adapting shared goals, they ensure their love story remains vibrant, relevant, and deeply fulfilling. Embracing the journey's fluidity, they create a tapestry of memories, dreams, and shared moments, proving that love, in its essence, is all about growing, evolving, and journeying together.

Chapter Seven

Intimacy and Physical Connection

"Intimacy is not purely physical. It's the act of connecting with someone so deeply, you feel like you can see into their soul." – Reshall Varsos

Intimacy is a multifaceted gem in the realm of relationships. Especially in age-gap dynamics, where the physical and emotional nuances might differ, understanding, navigating, and fostering intimacy becomes paramount. It's not just about the physical; it's about the profound bond, the silent conversations, the shared dreams, and the heartbeat synchronization. This section sheds light on the myriad dimensions of intimacy, offering insights and guidance for age-gap couples to nurture a profound, soul-deep connection.

1. The Depth Beyond Physicality:

- **Emotional intimacy**: Explore the realms of feelings, vulnerabilities, and dreams, building a connection that transcends the physical.

- **Intellectual intimacy**: Engage in stimulating conversations, debates, and mutual learning, forging a bond of minds.

- **Shared experiences**: Invest in activities that foster mutual growth, from traveling to art, creating a reservoir of shared memories.

2. Navigating Physical Differences:

- **Understanding age-related changes**: Delve into the physiological transformations with age, setting realistic expectations and fostering mutual understanding.

- **Staying active together**: Engage in physical activities as a couple, be it dancing, yoga, or hiking, to build stamina, synchronization, and mutual admiration.

- **Seeking medical advice**: Don't shy away from consulting professionals for any age-related physical concerns, ensuring a fulfilling physical relationship.

3. Rekindling the Passion:

- **Surprise elements**: Infuse the relationship with unexpected romantic gestures, from surprise dates to handwritten love notes.

- **Exploration**: Be open to exploring each other's desires and fantasies, ensuring mutual comfort and consent.

- **Intimacy rituals**: Create rituals, be it a specific song or a date night tradition, to keep the romantic spark alive.

4. Communication in Intimacy:

- **Open dialogues**: Foster an environment where both partners can discuss their desires, concerns, and boundaries without judgment.

- **Understanding non-verbal cues**: Learn to pick up on each other's unspoken signals, building a deeper connection.

- **Regular check-ins**: Periodically discuss the state of your intimate life, ensuring both partners are fulfilled and content.

5. Addressing Insecurities:

- **Positive affirmations**: Regularly reassure each other, focusing on the positives and strengths of the relationship.

- **Avoiding comparison**: Every relationship is unique. Steer clear of comparing your dynamic with others, embracing the beauty of your unique bond.

- **Seeking external support**: If insecurities become overwhelming, consider couples therapy or counseling for guidance and support.

Age-gap relationships, given their inherent differences, can offer a rich tapestry of intimate experiences. By focusing on mutual understanding, open communication, and shared growth, couples can build a bond that's both deeply emotional and passionately physical. After all, intimacy is about two souls dancing in harmony, creating a symphony that resonates through time.

***

Understanding Physical Changes with Age

Age is a profound journey of evolution, growth, and transformation. As the years roll by, the body undergoes various changes, some subtle and others more pronounced. In age-gap relationships, understanding and navigating these physical changes becomes essential to foster a loving, understanding, and fulfilling intimate connection. This section delves deep into the physiological metamorphoses that come with age and offers insights into how couples can gracefully navigate, adapt, and celebrate them.

Addressing Potential Health Challenges:

- **Being proactive**: Regular health check-ups and screenings are crucial to detect and address any potential health issues early on.

- **Open dialogues**: Foster a supportive environment where any health concerns or challenges can be discussed openly and without judgment.

- **Seeking professional guidance**: Engage with healthcare professionals to understand potential age-related health issues and their implications on intimacy.

Adapting to Differing Energy Levels:

- **Synchronized routines**: Try to align daily routines as much as possible, ensuring quality time together, despite differing energy peaks.

- **Mutual activities**: Engage in activities that cater to both partners' energy levels, such as leisurely walks, meditative practices, or rejuvenating spa sessions.

- **Understanding and patience**: Recognize and respect the natural ebbs and flows of energy in each other. This mutual understanding can pave the way for fulfilling intimate moments, tailored to both partners' comfort and enthusiasm levels.

Celebrating the Beauty of Mature Intimacy:

- **Deepening emotional connection**: Physical intimacy is enriched when coupled with emotional depth. Invest time in heartfelt conversations, shared dreams, and mutual vulnerabilities.

- **Exploring new avenues**: Age brings a depth of experience and wisdom. Explore new facets of intimacy that might not have been ventured into before, ensuring mutual comfort.

- **Cherishing the moments**: Recognize that every moment of intimacy is a celebration of the bond, the journey, and the shared life. Treasure these moments, seeing them as beautiful tapestries of love, trust, and mutual admiration.

Physical changes with age, while inevitable, need not be impediments. Instead, they can be avenues for growth, understanding, and deepened intimacy. By addressing challenges head-on, adapting with grace, and celebrating the profound beauty of mature intimacy, age-gap couples can craft a love story that's both passionate and deeply meaningful. In the dance of love, every step, every change, every beat is a testament to the journey shared.

***

Building Emotional Intimacy

In the vast expanse of human connection, emotional intimacy stands as a lighthouse, guiding the way to profound depths and uncharted terrains of the soul. It's more than just knowing a person; it's about understanding them, feeling them, and synchronizing with their heartbeat. Especially in age-gap relationships, where life experiences may differ significantly, building a bridge of emotional connection becomes pivotal. This section offers insights into nurturing this profound bond, turning it into the very bedrock of the relationship.

Deep Conversations and Shared Secrets:

- **Setting the stage**: Create a safe, cozy environment conducive to deep conversations—be it a late-night chat under the stars or a serene morning over coffee.

- **Venturing below the surface**: Move beyond mundane, everyday talk. Dive into philosophies, fears, passions, and memories. Share stories from the past, anecdotes from childhood, and musings about the universe.

- **Active listening**: Be truly present in these conversations. Listen with the heart, allowing the partner's words to resonate and echo within.

Building Trust and Vulnerability:

- **Consistency is key**: Trust is built brick by brick, through consistent actions, reliability, and integrity. Be someone your partner can always count on.

- **Open up**: Vulnerability is a two-way street. Open up about personal fears, insecurities, and dreams. This candidness encourages the partner to reciprocate, deepening the bond.

- **Respect boundaries**: Every individual has boundaries, some evident and some subtle. Recognize and respect these boundaries, ensuring they are never unintentionally crossed.

Exploring Mutual Dreams and Desires:

- **Dream mapping**: Spend an evening mapping out shared dreams, be it traveling to a particular destination, building a home, or writing a book together.

- **Collaborative ventures**: Engage in activities or projects that cater to mutual interests. This could range from taking a dance class, starting a joint blog, or gardening together.

- **Check-ins**: Regularly discuss and reassess shared goals and aspirations, ensuring both partners are aligned and excited about the journey ahead.

Emotional intimacy is a treasure trove of shared feelings, profound connections, and silent understandings. It's the warm hug on a cold night, the knowing glance across a crowded room, and the silent promise of forever. By fostering deep conversations, building unshakeable trust, and chasing shared dreams, age-gap couples can nurture a bond that stands the test of time, challenges, and the ever-evolving dance of life.

***

Navigating Physical Intimacy

Physical intimacy, a beautiful blend of passion, connection, and exploration, is an integral aspect of any romantic relationship. In age-gap romances, the differences in life experiences, bodily changes, and sometimes societal perceptions can add layers of complexity to this intimate dance. Yet, with understanding, communication, and a sprinkle of creativity, these very challenges can be transformed into avenues of deepened connection. This section offers guidance on embracing and enhancing physical intimacy, ensuring it remains a joyful, fulfilling aspect of the relationship.

Communicating Desires and Boundaries:

- **Open dialogues**: Create a safe space where both partners feel comfortable discussing their desires, fears, and limits without judgment.

- **Feedback loops**: Post-intimate moments, engage in gentle feedback sessions, discussing what felt great and what could be approached differently.

- **Continuous learning**: Relationships evolve, and so do desires. Regularly revisit conversations about physical intimacy, ensuring both partners feel heard and fulfilled.

Exploring Mutual Fantasies:

- **Dreamscape sessions**: Dedicate time to discuss and explore mutual fantasies, and understanding each other's deepest desires.

- **Safe experimentation**: Venture into new terrains of intimacy, always ensuring mutual consent and comfort. Remember, exploration is a journey, not a destination.

- **Resources and research**: Explore books, workshops, or couples' retreats centered on intimacy. This can provide fresh perspectives and ideas to incorporate into the relationship.

Overcoming Physical Challenges with Creativity:

- **Adapt and evolve**: If age-related physical challenges arise, view them as opportunities to innovate. For example, if stamina is an issue, focus on prolonged foreplay or intimate massages.

- **Professional guidance**: If physical issues persist, consider seeking guidance from a healthcare professional or therapist specializing in intimate relationships.

- **Celebrate connection**: Remember, intimacy isn't just about the physical act. Cherish the myriad ways you connect with your partner, be it through touch, words, or shared experiences.

Physical intimacy, while undeniably about passion, is equally about understanding, respect, and love. For age-gap couples willing to navigate the waters with empathy and creativity, the journey can be immensely fulfilling. By prioritizing open communication, exploring shared desires, and tackling challenges with a dash of innovation, they can craft a beautiful symphony of connection that resonates through the very core of their relationship.

***

Rekindling the Spark

Every relationship, no matter how passionate at the onset, can face moments where the flames seem to wane, where the spark feels a tad dimmer. This is a natural progression, and even more so in age-gap relationships where varying life stages can sometimes create distance. But the beauty lies in the ability to rekindle, to revisit the essence of what brought two souls together, and to fan those embers back into a roaring fire. This section dives into the art and heart of keeping the romance alive, ensuring that the journey, regardless of its length, remains as exhilarating as its start.

Planning Romantic Getaways:

- **Spontaneous escapades**: Sometimes, impromptu trips can rekindle passion like nothing else. Whisking away to a secluded beach or a charming countryside B&B can offer a respite from routine.

- **Memory lane trips**: Revisit places that hold special memories—where you first met, had your first date, or shared a significant moment. Reliving these memories can reawaken dormant emotions.

- **New adventures**: Chart unexplored territories together. Whether it's a hot air balloon ride, a trek through the wilderness, or a dance under the Northern Lights, novel experiences can reignite the thrill of discovery in the relationship.

Surprise Dates and Gestures:

- **Date night reinvention**: Surprise your partner with an elaborately planned date night. It could be a movie night at home with all their favorites or a reservation at that new restaurant they've been eager to try.

- **Small yet profound gestures**: Never underestimate the power of a handwritten note, a surprise gift, or even a spontaneous dance in the living room. These gestures, though seemingly small, can speak volumes.

- **Recreate firsts**: Re-enact your first date, your first kiss, or any other 'first' memory. These acts can remind both of you of the initial excitement and draw you closer.

Prioritizing Connection Amidst Busy Lives:

- **Sacred time blocks**: No matter how hectic life gets, earmark a fixed time daily or weekly for just the two of you—be it a morning coffee ritual or a nightly walk.

- **Digital detoxes**: In this age of omnipresent screens, periodically disconnecting from the digital world to connect with each other can be profoundly refreshing.

- **Active involvement**: Show genuine interest in each other's lives. Attend events or activities significant to your partner, ensuring they feel valued and cherished.

Love, in its purest form, is an ever-evolving dance of souls. And while the steps might sometimes falter, with conscious effort, understanding, and a sprinkling of romance, age-gap couples can ensure their dance remains as mesmerizing as the first sway. Through getaways, heartfelt gestures, and unwavering commitment, they can weave a tapestry of moments that not only rekindle the spark but set it ablaze with renewed passion.

Seeking External Support

Every relationship has its challenges, and while personal insight and mutual understanding can resolve many, seeking external perspectives can provide invaluable insights. Particularly for age-gap relationships, societal stigmas, coupled with the unique set of challenges they present, can sometimes necessitate a guiding hand to navigate tricky terrains. By actively seeking support, couples can bolster their bond, address underlying concerns, and fortify their relationship foundation.

Considering Couples Therapy:

- **Objective insights**: A neutral third-party perspective, like that of a therapist, can offer unbiased feedback and suggestions, helping couples address underlying issues they might be missing or avoiding.

- **Tools and techniques**: Therapists are trained to offer tools and strategies tailored to a couple's specific needs, assisting them in improving communication, understanding, and overall relationship health.

- **Safe space for tough conversations**: A therapeutic environment provides a non-judgmental space for couples to discuss deeper concerns, fears, or insecurities that might be challenging to broach otherwise.

Joining Support Groups for Age-Gap Relationships:

- **Shared experiences**: Meeting others in similar relationship dynamics can be comforting, offering a sense of camaraderie and understanding. Shared stories can also provide solutions to challenges one might be facing.

- **Building a community**: Support groups can help couples build a community of like-minded individuals, reducing feelings of isolation or "otherness" that might arise due to societal judgments.

- **Exchanging resources**: These groups often provide resources such as book recommendations, therapy contacts, or even group activities that cater specifically to age-gap couples, further fostering a sense of belonging.

Educating Oneself on Age-Related Physical Changes:

- **Understanding the biology**: By acquainting oneself with the natural physical changes that come with aging, couples can foster empathy and adjust expectations, ensuring a harmonious physical connection.

- **Adapting to changes**: Knowledge allows for adaptability. Understanding potential physical changes allows couples to find creative solutions, ensuring intimacy remains a strong pillar in the relationship.

- **Proactive health measures**: Being informed also means taking proactive steps in terms of health. This can range from regular medical check-ups, fitness regimes, or even dietary adaptations tailored to the older partner's needs.

Age-gap romances, with their unique blend of challenges and charms, can benefit immensely from external support. Whether it's the structured guidance of therapy, the community feel of support groups, or the empowerment of education, reaching out can often be the key to pulling closer together. Through these avenues, couples can deepen their understanding, cement their bond, and traverse their journey with renewed confidence and love.

Chapter Eight

Building Strong Foundations

"The best relationships are built on a foundation of respect and teamwork." – Unknown

Every lasting relationship is built on a foundation of trust, understanding, mutual respect, and shared goals. Age-gap relationships, given their unique dynamics, require a slightly nuanced approach to ensure these foundations are solid. This chapter delves into the foundational blocks crucial for the longevity of an age-gap romance, emphasizing the importance of a united front, common objectives, and mutual growth.

1. Trust and Honesty: The Cornerstones:

- **Open communication**: The significance of being honest about feelings, insecurities, and concerns, creating a transparent relationship environment.

- **Building reliability**: Ensuring both partners can count on each other, be it in small daily matters or significant life decisions.

- **Navigating jealousy and insecurities**: Age-gap relationships may occasionally be prone to doubts arising from the age difference; addressing these head-on is pivotal.

2. Shared Life Goals: Charting the Journey Together:

- **Clarifying aspirations**: Understanding each partner's dreams and desires, ensuring they are compatible or can be harmonized.

- **Short-term vs. long-term planning**: Emphasizing the importance of balancing immediate life plans with long-term aspirations.

- **Synchronizing timelines**: Given the age difference, ensuring major life milestones align or can be adjusted to suit both partners.

3. Building Mutual Respect:

- **Valuing differences**: Embracing the diversity in experiences, knowledge, and perspectives that each partner brings due to the age gap.

- **Avoiding patronizing behavior**: Ensuring the older partner does not inadvertently adopt a parent-like stance, and that both partners feel equal.

- **Honoring boundaries**: Recognizing and respecting personal and relational boundaries, ensuring neither partner feels suffocated or neglected.

4. Emotional Vulnerability and Support:

- **Being open about feelings**: The significance of letting guards down, allowing true feelings, fears, and dreams to be known.

- **Being each other's safe space**: Ensuring both partners feel they can turn to each other in times of distress, joy, or reflection.

- **Handling external pressures**: As age-gap relationships might face external skepticism, being each other's emotional anchor is crucial.

5. Continuous Growth and Adaptability:

- **Personal growth**: Recognizing that individual growth is vital for a relationship's health, and ensuring both partners continue to evolve and learn.

- **Growth as a couple**: Embracing new experiences, challenges, and joys together, further cementing the relationship bond.

- **Adapting to changes**: With age, life situations, health, and priorities can shift. Being adaptable ensures the relationship remains resilient through all phases.

Building a strong foundation is a conscious, continuous effort. It's about laying brick by brick, each representing trust, mutual respect, shared goals, and boundless love. With these foundations, age-gap relationships can thrive, proving that when love is true, numbers truly don't matter.

***

Trust is Paramount

Recognizing signs of a trustworthy partner:

- **Consistent Behavior**: A trustworthy partner's actions align with their words, creating a predictable and secure environment.

- **Openness**: They share their feelings, fears, and dreams transparently, allowing no room for unwarranted doubts.

- **Dependability**: Whether it's a promise or a casual commitment, they ensure they stick to their word, demonstrating reliability.

Building trust through actions:

- **Open Communication**: Engaging in candid conversations where feelings and concerns are freely expressed ensures misunderstandings are kept at bay.

- **Quality Time Together**: Building memories and sharing experiences adds layers to the trust foundation.

- **Integrity in Actions**: When actions mirror words consistently, trust is naturally fortified.

Rebuilding trust after challenges:

- **Acceptance**: Accepting the mistake and taking responsibility for the breach in trust is the first step to mending it.

- **Patient Listening**: Allowing the hurt partner to express their feelings without getting defensive ensures they feel valued.

- **Sustained Efforts**: Rebuilding trust isn't an overnight process. It requires time, patience, and consistent efforts to restore the relationship to its former glory.

In the world of age-gap romances, trust acts as the compass that guides partners through turbulent times and societal scrutiny. By understanding its importance, taking measures to foster it, and having the wisdom to mend it when broken, couples can ensure their relationship stands the test of time, proving love's transcendent nature over numbers.

***

Setting Boundaries

Recognizing personal boundaries:

- **Self-reflection**: Spend time understanding your own feelings, values, and what makes you uncomfortable or stressed. This helps in identifying boundaries that are essential for your well-being.

- **Listen to your instincts**: Your gut feeling is often a reliable guide. If something doesn't feel right or makes you uneasy, it's a cue that a boundary might be getting crossed.

- **Past experiences**: Reflecting on past relationships can give insights into what boundaries were lacking or which ones ensured a healthy relationship.

Communicating boundaries to your partner:

- **Clear and concise communication**: It's essential to be straightforward when communicating your boundaries. Avoid ambiguity to ensure your partner understands your perspective.

- **Choose the right moment**: Communicate when both of

you are calm and open to discussion. This ensures the conversation is productive and free from conflicts.

- **Use "I" statements**: Frame your needs using "I" statements like "I feel more comfortable when..." or "I need some time for...". This reduces blame and helps your partner understand it's about your needs.

Respecting and adhering to set boundaries:

- **Active listening**: When your partner communicates their boundaries, listen actively without getting defensive. This shows respect and understanding.

- **Avoid boundary testing**: Deliberately pushing or testing a partner's boundaries is a sign of disrespect. It's vital to steer clear of such behavior.

- **Regular check-ins**: Periodically revisit the boundaries discussion to see if they still hold or if any adjustments are needed based on changing circumstances or feelings.

Boundaries, far from being barriers, are actually the bridges that ensure each individual in the relationship can walk safely without infringing on the other's space. By recognizing, communicating, and respecting boundaries, age-gap couples can find the perfect balance where both partners coexist in harmony, understanding, and mutual respect.

***

The Power of Mutual Respect

Valuing each other's opinions and feelings:

- **Active Listening**: Ensure you give your partner undivided attention when they share. Listening shows you value their perspective, even if you don't always agree.

- **Acknowledge Differences**: Understand that coming from different generational backgrounds might mean varied opinions. Acknowledge these differences without belittling or dismissing them.

- **Encourage Expression**: Foster an environment where both of you feel safe expressing feelings, fears, and aspirations. This mutual openness amplifies respect.

Avoiding age-related power imbalances:

- **Be Conscious of Dynamics**: Recognize if age is being used as leverage in disagreements or decisions. Aim for equality rather than dominance.

- **Seek Feedback**: Regularly check in with your partner about how they feel regarding the power dynamics in the relationship. This helps in staying aware and making any necessary adjustments.

- **Equal Decision Making**: Ensure that major decisions, whether they concern finances, living arrangements, or future plans, are made jointly, honoring both perspectives.

Celebrating each other's strengths:

- **Acknowledge Achievements**: Celebrate each other's milestones, whether they're career-related, personal, or related to shared goals. Recognize the strengths that led to those achievements.

- **Lean on Each Other**: Recognize areas where your partner excels and seek their advice or support in those areas. This mutual leaning builds respect and showcases trust.

- **Shared Activities**: Engage in activities that allow both of you to showcase your strengths. It could be teaching each other something new, shared hobbies, or collaborative projects.

True respect goes beyond just surface-level politeness or adherence to societal norms. It delves deep into understanding, valuing, and cherishing each other's unique perspectives, strengths, and even vulnerabilities. In age-gap relationships, where external opinions can sometimes cloud judgment, holding onto this mutual respect can be the compass that always points toward love, understanding, and connection.

***

Investing in Relationship Growth

Prioritizing couple's activities and experiences:

- **Shared Adventures**: Whether it's traveling to a new destination, taking a class together, or exploring a shared hobby, shared experiences create lasting memories and strengthen the bond.

- **Routine Check-ins**: Set aside regular 'date nights' or 'relationship reviews' where you discuss the health of your relationship, celebrate achievements and address concerns.

- **Cultural Exchange**: Given the generational differences, introduce each other to movies, music, or events from your era. This not only bridges cultural gaps but also enriches the relationship.

Continuously learning about each other:

- **Deep Dive Conversations**: Every now and then, indulge in deep, meaningful conversations about dreams, fears, past experiences, or future aspirations.

- **Gift of Time**: Spend quality time together without distractions. This could be a quiet evening at home, a walk in the park, or even a weekend getaway.

- **Ask Open-Ended Questions**: Encourage conversations that allow both of you to explore and express freely by asking questions that don't have a simple 'yes' or 'no' answer.

Seeking mutual growth and evolution:

- **Personal Development**: Attend workshops or read books not just about relationships but also about personal growth. This ensures both partners are evolving, keeping the relationship fresh.

- **Feedback Loop**: Encourage a culture where both of you can give and receive feedback about the relationship, ensuring both partners are on the same page.

- **Shared Goals**: Set mutual short-term and long-term goals. This could relate to travel, financial planning, or even personal achievements. Working towards these together solidifies the partnership.

Relationships, much like living entities, need nourishment, care, and attention to flourish. In age-gap relationships, the investment in mutual growth ensures that the bond not only withstands the test of time but also becomes richer, deeper, and more rewarding with each passing day.

***

Dealing with External Influences

Navigating friendships and social circles:

- **Introducing the Partner**: Before introducing your older partner to your social circle, prepare both your friends and your partner for what to expect, highlighting common interests and setting the stage for pleasant interactions.

- **Choosing Social Events Wisely**: Recognize events or gatherings that are more likely to be accommodating and understanding, versus those that may put undue stress on your partner or the relationship.

- **Maintaining Individual Social Lives**: While it's important to integrate social circles, it's also crucial to have moments with your own friends, which can provide a respite and maintain individuality within the relationship.

Handling family dynamics and opinions:

- **Open Dialogue**: Address any family concerns head-on. Understand their worries while also explaining your perspective and the health of your relationship.

- **Pick Your Battles**: Not every comment or concern merits a response. Learn to distinguish between minor, ignorable issues and those that truly need addressing.

- **Seeking Mediation**: In cases where family resistance is strong, consider seeking family therapy or counseling to bridge understanding.

Balancing external influences with the relationship's core:

- **United Front**: Ensure that decisions regarding the relationship are made jointly. When faced with external pressures, present a united stance.

- **Setting Boundaries**: Clearly communicate to friends and family what topics or comments are off-limits. Over time, they'll learn to respect the relationship's boundaries.

- **Inner Circle**: Cultivate a close-knit circle of friends and family who truly understand and support the relationship. They can act as a buffer against negative external influences.

Remember, while the world may have an opinion, the true essence of a relationship is known only to the two people within it. By giving primacy to the relationship's core and addressing external influences with wisdom and grace, couples can build a foundation that stands strong amidst any storm.

***

Celebrating Age-Gap Love Stories

"Love knows not its own depth until the hour of separation." - Khalil Gibran

Age-gap relationships have been present throughout history and across cultures. They represent a special blend of wisdom, maturity, vigor, and freshness. This chapter aims to elevate the narrative around age-gap love stories by sharing some beautiful tales, both from history and from modern times, that exemplify the beauty and resilience of such relationships. Through these stories, readers can glean inspiration, hope, and affirmation.

1. Timeless Tales from History:

Anthony and Cleopatra:

- **Love over Power**: A romance that defied political pressures and ambitions.

- **Unified Front**: Their combined strengths challenged the might of Rome.

- **Legacy**: Their tale continues to inspire art, literature, and cinema.

Emmanuel Macron and Brigitte Trogneux:

- **Beyond Conventional Norms**: Emmanuel met Brigitte when he was a student and she, his teacher.

- **Support and Strength**: Despite societal scrutiny, Brigitte played a pivotal role in Emmanuel's presidential campaign.

- **Modern Role Models**: Their love story represents a modern validation of age-gap relationships.

2. Overcoming Challenges:

Lessons from Everyday Couples:

- **Dealing with Stigma**: Stories of couples who navigated societal pressures and came out stronger.

- **Facing Health Issues**: Inspiring tales of younger partners who supported their older counterparts through health challenges.

- **Embracing Parenting**: The joys and challenges of starting or extending a family in age-gap relationships.

3. Cultural Celebrations of Age-Gap Romances:

Literature and Movies:

- **Classic Literature**: Works like "The Graduate" and "Lolita" that touch upon age-gap themes.

- **Modern Films**: Celebrating movies like "The Age of Adaline" and "Harold and Maude" that portray the beauty of such relationships.

- **Evolution of Narratives**: How societal acceptance has shifted the portrayal of age-gap relationships in media over time.

4. Lessons from Successful Age-Gap Relationships:

Building Mutual Respect:

- **Prioritizing Communication**: How open dialogues have fortified relationships against external pressures.
- **Understanding Differences**: Celebrating stories where couples actively embraced their age-related differences.
- **Creating Shared Experiences**: Couples who've built bridges between their worlds to create a shared narrative.

5. Celebrating Your Own Story:

Creating Lasting Memories:

- **Documenting the Journey**: Keeping journals, taking photos, and cherishing moments together.
- **Revisiting Important Milestones**: Regularly celebrating

anniversaries, significant dates, and shared achievements.

- **Sharing with Others**: Using your own love story to inspire and encourage others in similar relationships.

In the end, age-gap relationships are just as valid, beautiful, and capable of enduring love as any other. By celebrating the rich tapestry of age-gap love stories from across the ages and from all walks of life, couples can find the inspiration and affirmation they need to cherish their own unique story.

***

Inspiring Age-Gap Love Stories

While age-gap relationships sometimes come under societal scrutiny, there are countless tales throughout history and in contemporary times that showcase the beauty, strength, and resilience of these unions. From historical figures who changed the course of events with their love, to modern-day celebrities who've shown that age is but a number, to personal stories that warm the heart – age-gap love is everywhere.

Historical Couples that Defied the Norms:
- **King Edward VIII and Wallis Simpson**:
  - **A King's Sacrifice**: Edward, who was 13 years younger than Wallis, abdicated his throne for the love they shared.

- **Media Scrutiny**: Their relationship was under constant media glare, yet they remained united.

- **Legacy**: A testament to the lengths one can go for love.

• **Augustus John and Dorelia McNeill**:

- **Bohemian Love**: The famed painter, 16 years Dorelia's senior, shared a deep bond with her, influencing his art.

- **Unconventional Union**: Living a non-traditional lifestyle, their love story became an inspiration for many.

- **Enduring Bond**: Despite challenges, their relationship lasted a lifetime.

Celebrity Relationships that Stood the Test of Time:

• **Michael Douglas and Catherine Zeta-Jones**:

- **Hollywood Royalty**: Despite the 25-year age difference, they've been one of Hollywood's most enduring couples.

- **Facing Challenges Together**: From health issues to career shifts, their unity remained unshaken.

- **Public Affection**: Their genuine affection and praise for one another in interviews are heartwarming.

• **Sarah Paulson and Holland Taylor**:

- **Defying Stereotypes**: With a 32-year age gap, these actresses have shown that love knows no bounds.

- **Supportive Partners**: They consistently uplift and celebrate each other's successes.

- **Advocates**: By being open about their relationship, they inspire others in age-gap unions.

Personal Stories of Age-Gap Success:

- **Anna & Roberto**:

  - **Meeting in Florence**: Anna, a student from the US, fell for Roberto, an Italian art historian, while studying abroad.

  - **Embracing Cultural Differences**: Navigating two cultures, they created a rich tapestry of shared experiences.

  - **Decades of Happiness**: Now grandparents, their story continues to inspire their community.

- **Evelyn & Tom**:

  - **Bonding Over Music**: Despite a 20-year age gap, Evelyn, a young jazz singer, and Tom, an established musician, created harmonies both on and off stage.

  - **Facing Doubters**: They proved skeptics wrong by building a strong foundation of trust and mutual respect.

  - **A Melodious Love**: Their love story became the stuff of local legend.

These age-gap love stories, spanning from history to the present day, are a testament to the enduring nature of love. They remind us that genuine connection and mutual respect are the cornerstones of any lasting relationship, regardless of age.

***

Challenges as Growth Opportunities

Every love story has its share of challenges, but for age-gap relationships, these challenges often come with an added layer of complexity. The silver lining? These unique challenges can become opportunities for deeper bonding, mutual growth, and an even stronger relationship foundation. Recognizing these moments not as pitfalls but as stepping stones is vital for nurturing a successful age-gap romance.

Viewing Difficulties as Bonding Experiences:

- **Shared Struggles**: Whether it's confronting societal judgment, navigating different life stages, or bridging cultural divides, facing these struggles together can cement the relationship.

- **Empathy & Understanding**: During trying times, the act of listening, understanding, and supporting can foster profound emotional closeness.

- **Creating a United Front**: Overcoming obstacles as a team enhances unity and mutual trust.

Recognizing the Strength in Overcoming Age-Related Challenges:

- **The Resilience Factor**: Age-gap couples often develop a resilience that becomes the backbone of their relationship, teaching them to face adversity head-on.

- **Unique Perspectives**: The beauty of different life experiences is that they provide unique perspectives, which, when combined, can offer a comprehensive view of any situation.

- **Validation Through Victory**: Every challenge surmounted together is a validation of the relationship's strength.

Celebrating Milestones and Successes:

- **Anniversaries & Achievements**: Every year together, every public acknowledgment, and every hurdle overcome should be celebrated as milestones in the relationship's journey.

- **Building a Memory Vault**: Creating and revisiting a collection of shared memories, be it through photos, journals, or shared experiences, can be a source of joy.

- **Public and Private Celebrations**: Whether it's a grand party with friends and family or a quiet evening reminiscing over wine, recognizing and reveling in the relationship's successes fosters positivity.

Understanding and embracing challenges as growth opportunities can transform age-gap relationships into a beacon of resilience, mutual respect, and lasting love. It's about rewriting the age-gap narrative and highlighting the beauty and strength inherent in such partnerships.

***

Creating Your Unique Love Story

Every age-gap relationship offers a chance to write a unique love story, distinct from any other. This chapter emphasizes the importance of documenting your journey, embracing shared goals, and weaving together an unforgettable narrative.

Building a Shared Narrative:

- **Melding Two Lives**: Combining two separate life histories into one cohesive story can be both challenging and beautiful. It requires understanding, patience, and mutual respect.

- **Recognizing Shared Moments**: Finding those key moments where your lives intersect and your stories overlap can solidify the bond.

- **Celebrating Differences**: Differences don't have to be divisive. Embracing the uniqueness of each partner can enhance the richness of the shared narrative.

Chronicling Your Journey Together:

- **Memory-Keeping**: Whether through scrapbooking, digital photo albums, or journaling, keeping a tangible record of shared experiences can be a treasured keepsake.

- **Documenting Milestones**: Big moments like vacations, anniversaries, or overcoming challenges should be celebrated and recorded.

- **Passing Down the Legacy**: Sharing your love story with future generations can be a way of leaving behind a lasting legacy of love, understanding, and resilience.

Setting Goals and Dreams as a Couple:

- **Dreaming Together**: Whether it's traveling to a dream destination, buying a home, or simply planning for retirement, shared dreams can act as anchors in the relationship.

- **Mapping Out the Journey**: Planning together for the realization of these dreams ensures both partners are invested and on the same page.

- **Adapting and Evolving**: Dreams may change with time, and being flexible and understanding can ensure the relationship remains strong and fulfilling.

Creating your unique love story isn't just about documenting the past; it's about planning for the future, celebrating the present, and cherishing every moment spent together. This intentional celebration of shared experiences can be the foundation of a lasting, loving relationship.

***

Supporting Others in Age-Gap Relationships

Age-gap relationships can offer rich insights into love, trust, and understanding. But like any other form of relationship, they come with their challenges. By offering support and sharing experiences, we can lift up others in similar relationships, creating a community where love transcends numbers.

Building Communities and Support Groups:

- **Local Initiatives**: Encourage and start local support groups where age-gap couples can meet, share, and bond over common experiences.

- **Online Forums**: The digital age offers a plethora of platforms where couples can connect across distances, fostering global connections.

- **Organizing Workshops**: By hosting or attending seminars focusing on age-gap relationships, couples can gather a wealth of knowledge and strategies to strengthen their bond.

Sharing Experiences and Advice:

- **Narratives of Love**: Sharing personal stories can be therapeutic and can offer others in similar situations solace and guidance.

- **Publishing Resources**: Be it books, blogs, or podcasts, creating resources can provide lasting advice and insights for age-gap couples.

- **Open Dialogues**: Regularly hosting or attending sessions where couples discuss challenges and solutions can pave the way for deeper understanding and stronger bonds.

Uplifting Others Through Shared Wisdom:

- **Mentorship Programs**: Couples who have successfully navigated their age-gap journey can offer invaluable guidance to those newer to the experience.

- **Celebrate Love**: Organizing events where couples celebrate their milestones can boost morale and offer a sense of community.

- **Promote Inclusivity**: By fostering environments that are free of prejudice and rich in understanding, we can ensure that every age-gap couple feels seen, heard, and valued.

In the end, by lifting each other up and sharing our journeys, age-gap couples can create a world that not only accepts but celebrates their unique love story.

***

Looking Forward with Hope

Every relationship, regardless of age differences, has its highs and lows. Yet, the allure and depth found in age-gap romances provide couples with a unique tapestry of experiences. As with all things, looking forward with hope can illuminate the path even during challenging times, ensuring that the love story continues to evolve beautifully.

Envisioning a Future Filled with Love:

- **Shared Dreams**: Mapping out mutual aspirations and dreams as a couple can provide direction and purpose.

- **Moments of Reflection**: Regularly reminiscing about shared experiences can deepen the bond and keep the spark alive.

- **Continual Growth**: Actively seeking opportunities to grow together, both personally and as a couple, ensures a dynamic and evolving relationship.

Navigating Challenges with Optimism:

- **Positive Reinforcement**: Celebrating small wins and achievements can foster a culture of positivity and resilience.

- **Seeking External Counsel**: Whether it's through therapy or counseling, gaining an external perspective can offer new strategies and insights.

- **Mindset Shift**: By framing challenges as opportunities rather than setbacks, couples can navigate through tough times with a solution-oriented mindset.

Cherishing the Beauty of Age-Gap Romance:

- **Unique Dynamics**: Appreciating the unique blend of maturity and freshness that age-gap couples bring to a relationship.

- **Collective Wisdom**: The combination of experiences from different life stages can offer a profound depth to the relationship.

- **Timeless Romance**: Recognizing that true love isn't bound by age, and celebrating the ageless nature of love in all its forms.

The journey of age-gap romance, filled with its unique nuances, provides an enriching narrative of love that transcends time. By looking forward with hope and cherishing each moment, couples can build a legacy of love that stands the test of time.

Chapter Nine

Celebrating Age-Gap Love Stories

"Love knows no age. Real love isn't about being with someone who meets a certain criteria, it's about being with someone who makes you feel a certain way." – Unknown

Age-gap relationships, while unique in their dynamics, are as rich and profound as any love story. Through the passage of time, many such relationships have inspired, faced challenges, and yet emerged strong, leaving behind tales of unparalleled love. In this chapter, let's delve into and celebrate these stories that transcend age, time, and often, societal norms.

1. Inspiring Age-Gap Love Stories:

- **Historical Legends**: Tales from history that showcase age-gap relationships defying societal expectations and flouruishing.

- **Modern-Day Icons**: Celebrity age-gap relationships that have inspired and given hope to many, showing that love knows no age.

- **Real-Life Tales**: Personal narratives from everyday individuals who found love where age wasn't a factor but compatibility was.

2. Challenges as Growth Opportunities:

- **Strength in Adversity**: How challenges unique to age-gap relationships often lead to deeper understanding and stronger bonds.

- **Milestones Worth Celebrating**: The joy of overcoming prejudices and misconceptions, and milestones that deserve celebration.

- **Learning & Growing Together**: Embracing differences, learning from each other's life experiences, and evolving together.

3. Creating Your Unique Love Story:

- **Crafting A Shared Journey**: Building shared experiences and memories that define the relationship.

- **Cherishing Personal Moments**: Celebrating small, personal moments that may seem insignificant but form the crux of the relationship.

- **Dreaming Together**: Envisioning a shared future and working towards it, regardless of age.

4. Supporting Others in Age-Gap Relationships:

- **Building A Supportive Community**: The importance of creating safe spaces and communities for age-gap couples to share, discuss, and support.

- **Sharing Wisdom**: Offering insights, experiences, and lessons to others navigating similar relationships.

- **Being Allies**: Standing up against prejudices and misconceptions, and advocating for age-gap relationships.

5. Looking Forward with Hope:

- **Evolving Together**: Continuously adapting, changing, and growing with each other, cherishing every stage of life.

- **Being Torchbearers**: Representing hope and strength for future age-gap couples, leading by example.

- **Embracing The Future**: Moving ahead with optimism, knowing that the foundation is love, understanding, and mutual respect.

In celebrating age-gap love stories, we celebrate the indomitable spirit of love itself, which remains unfazed by time or age. The essence of such relationships lies in understanding, mutual respect, and the shared experiences that knit two souls together, proving time and again that love, truly, knows no bounds.

***

Inspiring Age-Gap Love Stories

In the world of romance, where the heart leads, the years often take a backseat. Love stories that transcend age differences have existed throughout history, continue to capture the public's imagination in the modern day, and manifest quietly in everyday lives. Such relationships, with all their unique challenges and beauty, are a testament to the idea that love knows no boundaries. Let's explore these relationships, from history's annals to the silver screen, and even in the homes next door.

Historical couples that defied the norms:
- **Cleopatra and Julius Caesar**: An iconic relationship that not only spanned age differences but also cultures and empires. Their love story is emblematic of power, intrigue, and passion.

- **Emperor Shah Jahan and Mumtaz Mahal**: Beyond the majestic Taj Mahal, a symbol of undying love, lies the story of a profound age-gap romance that has left an indelible mark on history.

- **Dante and Beatrice**: Though not traditionally a couple, Dante's admiration and love for Beatrice, who was younger, inspired much of his work, showing the depth of his feelings.

Celebrity relationships that stood the test of time:
- **Michael Douglas and Catherine Zeta-Jones**: With an age difference of 25 years, their relationship has withstood Hollywood pressures, health challenges, and more, proving that age-gap relationships can endure.

- **Hugh Jackman and Deborra-Lee Furness**: Their love story breaks conventional norms, with Furness being 13 years older than Jackman. They've been together for decades, continuously defying critics.

- **Sarah Paulson and Holland Taylor**: An inspiring couple that not only navigates an age gap but also challenges in the LGBTQ+ community, showcasing their strength and commitment to one another.

Personal stories of age-gap success:
- **Ella and Sam**: Met in a book club, with a 20-year difference between them. Their shared love for literature and mutual respect has cemented their relationship, proving that interests often transcend age.

- **Nina and Greg**: Despite a 15-year age difference, their mutual passion for traveling has taken them on numerous adventures together, strengthening their bond.

- **Sophie and Richard**: With an age gap of 30 years, their relationship faced skepticism. Yet, their mutual goals, trust, and love for music helped them craft a beautiful life together, illustrating that age is but a number when two souls connect.

Each of these stories, be it from history, Hollywood, or home, underscores the sentiment that age-gap relationships are not just about the years between two people, but the shared moments, trust, understanding, and love that binds them. They teach us that in the realm of love, age truly becomes secondary to connection, respect, and shared dreams.

***

Challenges as Growth Opportunities

Every relationship encounters hurdles, and those with an age gap might face a unique set of them. Yet, it's these very challenges that often become the foundation of the strongest bonds, molding the relationship into something even more special. When faced with adversity, age-gap couples have the opportunity to use these moments as growth opportunities, turning difficulties into enduring love stories.

Viewing difficulties as bonding experiences:
- **The Stigma Challenge**: Society, unfortunately, sometimes casts a skeptical eye on age-gap relationships. But for many couples, these challenges have acted as a crucible, solidifying their bond. Facing the world together, defending their love, they learn to rely on one another, forging a bond that's often unbreakable.

- **Different Life Stages**: When one partner is in their career's prime while the other is considering retirement, or when one wishes to start a family while the other has adult children, these are not just challenges but moments that demand understanding and compromise. Through these, couples learn the art of sacrifice, adjustment, and the depth of their commitment to one another.

Recognizing the strength in overcoming age-related challenges:
- **Health Concerns**: With age might come health issues. In such moments, the younger partner often steps into the role of caregiver, showcasing a depth of love and commitment that's profound.

- **Cultural Gaps**: Whether it's a favorite song from the '60s or the latest viral trend, navigating cultural differences requires patience. Over time, couples find joy in introducing each other to their worlds, be it old-school classics or the newest tech gadget.

Celebrating milestones and successes:
- **Anniversaries**: Every year marks not just another year together but the triumph over the challenges faced. These moments become even more precious, a testament to their enduring love.

- **Achieving Mutual Goals**: Be it traveling to a dream destination, buying a home, or even simpler joys like mastering a recipe together – these milestones, achieved together, are moments of shared pride.

- **Overcoming Prejudices**: Every time a skeptic turns into a supporter, every time a doubting friend sees the love and becomes an ally, it's a victory, a celebration of their love's authenticity.

In the end, challenges aren't barriers; they are stepping stones. For couples with an age difference, each hurdle overcome is a testament to their resilience, their commitment, and the timeless nature of their love. The beauty lies not in a life without challenges but in a love that overcomes them.

***

Creating Your Unique Love Story

Introduction: Every love story is unique, and age-gap romances have their special charm and set of experiences. It's not just about the number of years that set you apart, but the multitude of shared experiences, mutual respect, and dreams that bind you together. Crafting your unique narrative is a conscious effort, filled with cherished memories, shared dreams, and a roadmap of the journey you wish to take together.

Building a shared narrative:
- **Melding Two Worlds**: The beauty of age-gap relationships often lies in the melding of two different worlds. It's about creating a new world together, where memories from the past and dreams of the future coexist harmoniously. Every movie night with films from different decades, every shared

story of childhood, contributes to this shared narrative.

- **Establishing Traditions**: Whether it's an annual trip to a favorite place, cooking a meal from each other's childhood, or just a simple ritual like a morning walk - these become threads that weave your unique love story.

- **Handling Challenges Together**: Every hurdle, every skeptic faced, and every challenge overcome become chapters in your love story, proving the strength of your bond.

Chronicling your journey together:
- **Photo Albums and Journals**: In the digital age, there's a unique charm in maintaining physical photo albums or writing journals. They can be a tangible testament to your journey, filled with annotated memories, ticket stubs, and notes.

- **Digital Memories**: Creating shared blogs, vlogs, or even private digital spaces where you document your experiences can be a modern take on chronicling your love.

- **Legacy Projects**: Whether it's a tree you plant together or a business you start, projects that outlive the moment and carry forward your combined legacy can be a powerful way of documenting your journey.

Setting goals and dreams as a couple:
- **Short-term Goals**: These could range from simple objectives like taking a dance class together, visiting a new city, or achieving a financial target.

- **Long-term Dreams**: From where you see yourselves in the next decade, retirement plans, or even philanthropic ventures – these dreams give direction to your shared journey.

- **Reassessing Periodically**: As with any relationship, dreams and goals can evolve. Regular check-ins ensure that both partners are on the same page and any new dreams are incorporated into the shared vision.

Your love story isn't just defined by the age difference but by the countless moments, big and small, that you experience together. It's a constantly evolving tapestry of memories, dreams, challenges, and triumphs – a unique narrative that only the two of you can craft.

***

Supporting Others in Age-Gap Relationships

Introduction: Navigating the intricacies of age-gap relationships can be a solitary journey, especially in a world that often misunderstands or stigmatizes such unions. However, there's a unique strength in the community. By creating spaces where others can share their experiences, seek advice, and find validation, couples can give back to the age-gap community and pave the way for more understanding and acceptance.

Building communities and support groups:
- **Initiating Safe Spaces**: Start by creating online forums or local meetup groups specifically geared towards age-gap couples. Safe spaces like these can help individuals share

their stories, find friends in similar relationships, and derive strength from collective experiences.

- **Collaborative Activities**: Organize events, workshops, or retreats that focus on building relationships, improving communication, and celebrating the uniqueness of age-gap love stories. This could include couples' therapy sessions, movie nights featuring age-gap love stories, or book clubs reading relevant literature.

- **Advocacy and Awareness**: As a community, take steps to challenge stereotypes and promote a more inclusive view of love. This could be done through creating content, hosting seminars, or collaborating with influencers who resonate with the age-gap narrative.

Sharing experiences and advice:
- **Guest Speaking and Panels**: Hosting or participating in panels and discussions about age-gap relationships can bring visibility to real-life experiences.

- **Blogs and Vlogs**: Documenting your journey and sharing advice on platforms like blogs, YouTube, or even podcasts can provide invaluable insights to those new to the age-gap relationship world.

- **Mentoring**: Consider mentoring newer age-gap couples who might be struggling with challenges you've already navigated. Your experiences could provide comfort and guidance.

Uplifting others through shared wisdom:

- **Celebrating Success Stories**: Sharing testimonials and success stories can be a beacon of hope for many. It demonstrates the resilience and depth of age-gap relationships.

- **Resource Sharing**: Compile resources – be it books, articles, or counseling services – that have helped you in your journey. Sharing these can provide a solid foundation for others.

- **Affirmations and Encouragement**: Sometimes, a simple word of encouragement can make all the difference. Be an active source of positivity in the community, reminding others of the beauty and strength inherent in their unique love stories.

By taking a proactive role in supporting others, you not only strengthen the community but also fortify your own relationship. There's power in numbers, and as more couples come together, the message becomes clear: Love isn't bound by age; it's defined by understanding, respect, and shared experiences.

***

Supporting Others in Age-Gap Relationships

Introduction: Navigating the intricacies of age-gap relationships can be a solitary journey, especially in a world that often misunderstands or stigmatizes such unions. However, there's a unique strength in the community. By creating spaces where others can share their experiences, seek advice, and find validation, couples can give back to the age-gap community and pave the way for more understanding and acceptance.

Building communities and support groups:
- **Initiating Safe Spaces**: Start by creating online forums or local meetup groups specifically geared towards age-gap couples. Safe spaces like these can help individuals share their stories, find friends in similar relationships, and derive strength from collective experiences.

- **Collaborative Activities**: Organize events, workshops, or retreats that focus on building relationships, improving communication, and celebrating the uniqueness of age-gap love stories. This could include couples' therapy sessions, movie nights featuring age-gap love stories, or book clubs reading relevant literature.

- **Advocacy and Awareness**: As a community, take steps to challenge stereotypes and promote a more inclusive view of love. This could be done through creating content, hosting seminars, or collaborating with influencers who resonate with the age-gap narrative.

Sharing experiences and advice:
- **Guest Speaking and Panels**: Hosting or participating in panels and discussions about age-gap relationships can bring visibility to real-life experiences.

- **Blogs and Vlogs**: Documenting your journey and sharing advice on platforms like blogs, YouTube, or even podcasts can provide invaluable insights to those new to the age-gap relationship world.

- **Mentoring**: Consider mentoring newer age-gap couples who might be struggling with challenges you've already navigated. Your experiences could provide comfort and guidance.

Uplifting others through shared wisdom:
- **Celebrating Success Stories**: Sharing testimonials and success stories can be a beacon of hope for many. It demonstrates the resilience and depth of age-gap relationships.

- **Resource Sharing**: Compile resources – be it books, articles, or counseling services – that have helped you in your journey. Sharing these can provide a solid foundation for others.

- **Affirmations and Encouragement**: Sometimes, a simple word of encouragement can make all the difference. Be an active source of positivity in the community, reminding others of the beauty and strength inherent in their unique love stories.

By taking a proactive role in supporting others, you not only strengthen the community but also fortify your own relationship. There's power in numbers, and as more couples come together, the message becomes clear: Love isn't bound by age; it's defined by understanding, respect, and shared experiences.

***

Looking Forward with Hope

Introduction: In the journey of age-gap relationships, hope acts as a guiding star, illuminating the path through uncertainties and challenges. Embracing a hopeful perspective not only nurtures the relationship but also equips couples to envision a brighter, love-filled future. Let's delve into the facets of maintaining this hope and cherishing the distinctive beauty of age-gap romance.

Envisioning a future filled with love:

- **Dream Together**: Engage in regular discussions about your collective future. This can range from picturing your ideal home, planning trips you'd love to take, or visualizing family gatherings in years to come.

- **Set Tangible Goals**: Whether it's buying a home together, adopting a pet, or traveling to a dream destination, setting tangible goals brings dreams to life and strengthens the bond.

- **Celebrate Achievements**: Mark milestones, both big and small. Commemorate anniversaries, celebrate each other's accomplishments, and cherish the everyday moments that make your love story unique.

Navigating challenges with optimism:

- **Reframe Perspectives**: When faced with challenges, focus on the lessons and growth opportunities they present. Viewing obstacles as stepping stones to a stronger relationship can transform your approach to them.

- **Cultivate Resilience**: Remind each other of past challenges you've overcome as a team. This collective memory acts as a testament to your resilience and capability.

- **Seek Inspiration**: Draw inspiration from other age-gap couples, literature, movies, or any source that resonates with your narrative. Witnessing others navigate similar paths with grace can instill confidence in your journey.

Cherishing the beauty of age-gap romance:
- **Embrace Differences**: Celebrate the unique blend of experiences, perspectives, and wisdom that an age-gap brings to the table. These differences enrich your shared story.

- **Create Traditions**: Establish rituals or traditions that capture the essence of your relationship. It could be as simple as watching a classic movie from each other's generation or reading together each night.

- **Reflect and Appreciate**: Regularly take moments to reflect on your journey. Appreciate the depths, the highs, the challenges, and the love that has held you together. Such reflections deepen gratitude and renew passion.

Looking forward with hope isn't just a passive expectation; it's an active endeavor. By nurturing this mindset, age-gap couples can create a love story that not only endures but thrives, standing as a testament to the timeless nature of love, irrespective of age.

Chapter Ten

Conclusion

Reflecting on the Journey: The Beauty and Challenges of Age-Gap Romance:
Age-gap romances, like all love stories, are an amalgamation of shared memories, heartwarming moments, challenges, and growth. The unique blend of experiences and perspectives that both partners bring adds a distinct color and texture to their shared narrative. While age-gap couples might face challenges that are specific to their situation, their journey stands testament to the timelessness of love, proving that the heart knows no age. It's a dance of two souls intertwined, where age merely adds layers of depth, wisdom, and understanding to the relationship.

Embracing Love in All Its Forms: Celebrating Diverse Relationships:
Love, in its myriad forms and expressions, remains one of the most powerful and universal emotions. Whether it's an age-gap relationship, same-age romance, or any other form of bond, every relationship tells a unique story. In a world rich with diversity, it's essential to celebrate and respect love in all its avatars. Age-gap romances teach us that love isn't bound by societal norms or expectations; it's an ever-evolving

emotion that finds its way, regardless of age, cultural background, or life experiences.

A Call to Action: Building a Lasting and Fulfilling Age-Gap Relationship:

For those embarking on or navigating the waters of an age-gap relationship, the journey might be filled with unique challenges. Yet, as we've explored, it's also brimming with unparalleled beauty and growth opportunities. Take heart in knowing that every relationship requires work, understanding, and commitment. Use the insights and strategies shared in this guide as a compass. Continue to learn, grow, and evolve with your partner.

Remember, the foundation of any lasting relationship is trust, mutual respect, and love. Keep these principles at the heart of your age-gap romance, and you'll weave a love story that stands the test of time. Love, in all its glory and complexity, is a journey worth embarking upon. Here's to building and cherishing a fulfilling age-gap relationship that's uniquely yours.

www.ingramcontent.com/pod-product-compliance
Lightning Source LLC
LaVergne TN
LVHW021828060526
838201LV00058B/3555